Speed and Efficiency: Demystifying Next-Generation Sequencing Technology

Nain

Contents

4 Data integration in NGS   56

5 Functional characterisation of long non-coding RNAs   79

6 General discussion and conclusions   113

Chapter 1

Introduction

1.1   Next Generation Sequencing

Next generation sequencing (NGS) technologies have revolutionised the way genomics and molecular biology research has been carried out during this last decade. The advent of these "new" technologies has allowed researchers to sequence complete genomes much faster and cheaper compared to the old Sanger sequencing, making them much more affordable for researchers (Figure 1.1).

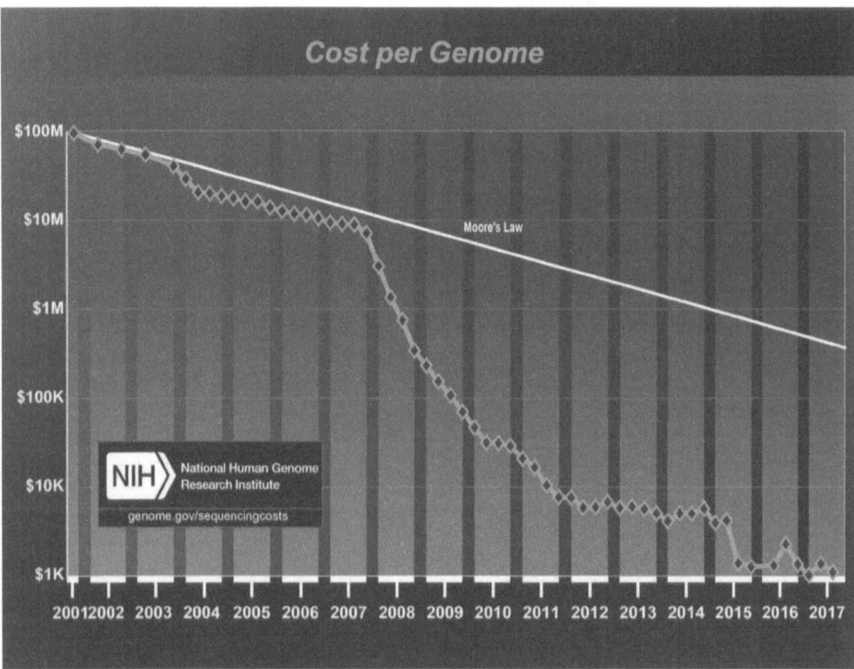

Figure 1.1: Evolution of whole human genome sequencing cost over the years. Courtesy: National Human Genome Research Institute.

The human genome is composed of more than 3 billion base pairs. Current sequencing reactions can only cover a fraction of hundreds of base pairs at a time. This means that in order to cover the whole human genome, thousands of overlapping slices of DNA sequence need to be produced. NGS uses massively parallel sequencing to generate millions of reads of data simultaneously. Generally, a typical NGS workflow includes the following steps: the DNA is randomly fragmented, the resulting segments are size-selected and adapters are ligated to both 5' and 3' ends. The sequence generation step occurs differently depending on the platform [1]: fragments are attached to a solid surface on Illumina, where sequencing occurs. In the Pacbio platform, sequencing happens in a zero-wavelength chamber and in SOLiD, inside a droplet. In the case of Nanopore, the protagonists are the pores, and sequencing happens as the DNA molecules pass through. Data in the form of nucleotides is obtained after processing the raw signals, which are specific for each platform. The advantage of these technologies and one of the main differences compared to the Sanger sequencing is the opportunity to perform the final sequencing step simultaneously for an entire library of DNA fragments.

1.1.1 Sequencing platforms

The first sequencer, 454, was introduced in 2005 by Roche and it was rapidly followed in 2006 by two other platforms: SOLiD (Life Technologies) and Solexa (Illumina). Each platform used a different approach for sequencing, leading to different results in regards to throughput (i.e. number of reads, read length), signal to noise detection, run time and, equally important, final cost. 454 relied on beads as the solid surface where adaptor-ligated single-stranded fragments were joined (one fragment per bead) and amplified in an emulsion PCR. Amplified beads were immobilised in a multi-well plate or a glass slide, where the sequencing reaction occurred via pyrosequencing. In this method, additional beads with a sulphurylase and a luciferase were introduced to react with the pyrophosphate released by the last incorporated base, generating ATP, which reacts with luciferin producing oxyluciferin and light. This light was monitored and the signals translated into a sequence. This platform was mostly used to perform *de novo* sequencing of bacteria and organisms of low complexity, some exome analysis and 16S metagenomics [1], although its use was discontinued in 2016.

SOLiD sequencing, instead, used a different approached called sequencing by ligation. The workflow also included an emulsion PCR on beads, however, the sequencing was performed using several ligation rounds where fluorescently labelled di-base probes competed for ligation to the sequencing primer or the previous probe. After five rounds, the complete sequence of each fragment was obtained. One of the main advantages of SOLiD versus the 454 platform was its ability to better sequence homopolymers and repeat regions as well as having higher throughput. SOLiD was more often applied to variant discovery through re-sequencing projects [1].

But, without any doubt, the platform that revolutionised the field was Illumina, with a sequencing methodology called solid-phase amplification. Briefly, sheared single-stranded DNA fragments linked to adaptors are hybridised into a solid surface coated with forward and reverse primers. The adaptors on the attached DNA segments can ligate to nearby complementary attached oligonucleotides forming a bridge. Fluorescently-labelled nucleotides are added in several rounds, so that a PCR is performed in each of these bridges, forming a cluster of identical sequences. The incorporation of each nucleotide includes the release of a fluorescent signal, which is captured by an imaging system. Post-sequencing management of these images reveals the complete sequence of each cluster/fragment. The use of the Illumina platform is still on the rise worldwide, and its applications have been very broad, i.e., variant discovery, exome sequencing and gene discovery [1]. Comparatively, 454 was able to produce longer reads (400-600 million bp per run with 400-500 bp read lengths), however, the quality and throughput were very low compared to SOLiD and Illumina, and the error rate higher. SOLiD, on its side, provided high throughput but with very small reads (2.8 billion 50-75 bp paired-end reads). Strikingly, Illumina HiSeq can now produce 5 billion 150 bp paired-reads per run, and the latest Novaseq, up to 20 billion. A structure that includes 10 Illumina HiSeq machines (HiSeq X Ten) can yield nearly 3 billion paired-end 150-bp sequences. This is the sequencer that broke the $1000 barrier to perform whole-genome sequencing of the human genome. Other platforms were also commercialised: the Ion Torrent (Life Technologies, 2010) was promising as a bench-top device with a different sequencing strategy based on monitoring pH changes caused by the incorporation of a new nucleotide into the growing strand. However, a new revolution took place in the field by the introduction of the single-molecule real-time (SMRT) sequencing. No amplification reaction is performed in these cases, avoiding the inherent bias caused by this process. In 2011, the Pac-Bio RS system (Pacific Biosciences) was released as the first one capable of performing direct SMRT sequencing using immobilised polymerase enzymes. Three years later, Oxford Nanopore Technologies (ONT) released the MinION, the first portable sequencer that identifies DNA bases by measuring changes in the electrical conductivity of a membrane as the DNA passes through a biological pore. ONT recently released the GridION as a scalable sequencer using the same approach. These two platforms produce long reads, which in the case of PacBio can reach an average of 10kb (maximum length 60 kb), while ONT technologies can surpass the 150kb. The revolution of long-read sequencing has occurred mainly in the field of microbial genomics and real-time pathogen identification [2, 3]. The main advantage of long-read sequencing is the ability to deal with complex genomic regions and structural variants, allowing to resolve complex areas of the human genome as well as lower-complexity organisms [4]. Very recently, the portable MinION device was used to sequence the whole human genome with a 30x depth, achieving almost 86% coverage of the reference GRCh38 sequence, with a great improvement in the assembly of the major histocompatibility complex, telomere repeats and closing existing gaps [5].

All these platforms differ in the chemistry and processing steps. Their final output data (raw data) can have a platform-dependent format, however, all of them currently provide a conversion to the so-called *fastq* file. This file is usually the starting point for any current bioinformatics pipeline.

1.2   General pipeline in NGS

Figure 1.2 shows a typical NGS pipeline. *Fastq* files are no more than text files containing 4 lines per sequenced fragment or read (the read id, the nucleotide sequence, an optional id or description and the sequence of encoded qualities for each nucleotide). This format has become the standard, so NGS platforms either generate these files directly or generates a different file format that can be converted to *.fastq*.

```
@SEQUENCE_ID
GATTTGGGGTTCAAAGCAGTATCGATCAAATAGTAAATCCATTTGTTCAACTCACAGTTT
+
!''*(((((***+))%%%++)(%%%%).1***-+*''))**55CCF>>>>>>CCCCCCC65
```

Fastq quality scores are ASCII-encoded and are commonly referred to as *Phred Quality Scores*, which measure the probability of a base being incorrectly called. For example, a quality score of 10 would mean that there is a probability of 1 in 10 that the base call is incorrect (90% accuracy), while a value of 50 would mean there is a probability of 1 in 100000 to be incorrect (99.999% accuracy).

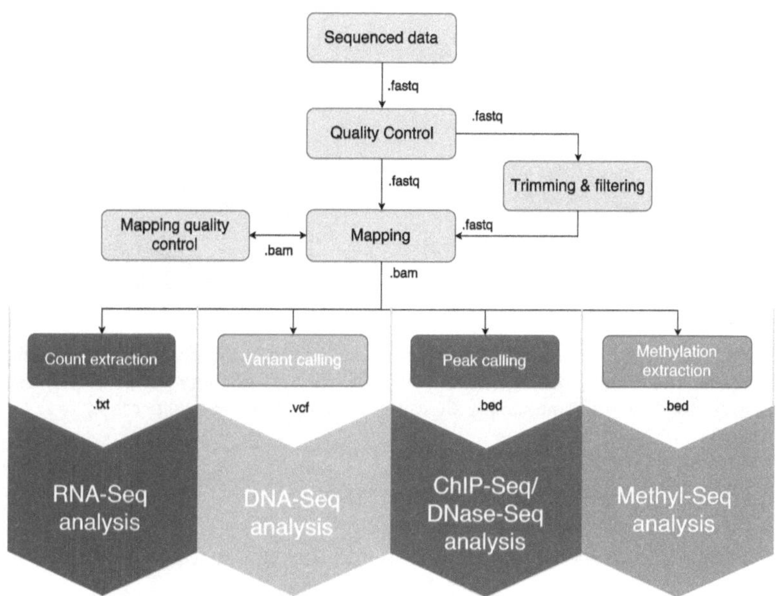

Figure 1.2: General bioinformatics pipeline in NGS experiments.

1.2.1 Quality Control (QC) of the data

First, quality control of the reads should be performed to discard those reads or segments of reads with poor qualities. A typical threshold would be to keep all the reads with Phred Quality Scores over 30 (99.9% accuracy). While programs such as FastQC [6] can help to get an overview of the quality of the sequences and discover different types of biases, some tools from the FASTX-Toolkit [`http://hannonlab.cshl.edu/fastx_toolkit/`] or such as cutadapt [7] allow filtering out or trimming reads based on some quality conditions as well as remove known adapter sequences from the reads. An example of the results of cleaning can be seen in Figure 1.3.

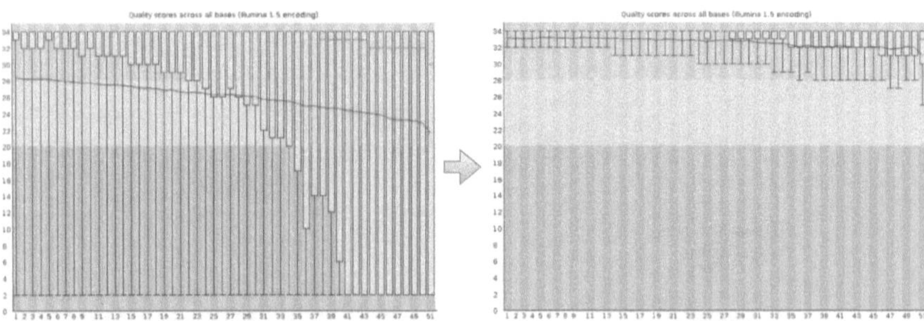

Figure 1.3: Quality score across all the bases of a sample FastQ file before and after cleaning low quality reads. The first figure shows a sample containing reads of very low quality. The second figure corresponds to the same sample after filtering out those low-quality reads.

1.2.2   *Reference mapping and de novo assembly*

Once all the reads pass the quality thresholds, they are ready for subsequent analyses. Depending on the aim of the project, reads can be assembled to each other (*de novo* assembly) or mapped to a reference genome (mapping). A *de novo* assembly is generally performed when the genome being studied has not been characterised yet. This is a hard process that requires high sequencing depth and read quality. The algorithm (i.e. de Bruijn graph [8]) tries to reconstruct the whole genome by overlapping reads to each other to form contigs. The main output, in this case, corresponds to a *fasta* file containing the sequence of these contigs. On the other hand, if the reference genome is already known, it can be used as a guide to overlap the reads. This method allows identifying the chromosome position where the read fragment was sequenced. Not all the reads will map to the reference genome because of potential sequencing errors or differences between the sample and the reference genome sequences. In the same way, not all the input reads will be used for the final *de novo* assembly. In the mapping process, the output file will be in SAM or BAM (the binary format of SAM) format. A SAM file is a plain text file containing the sections from Figure 1.4:

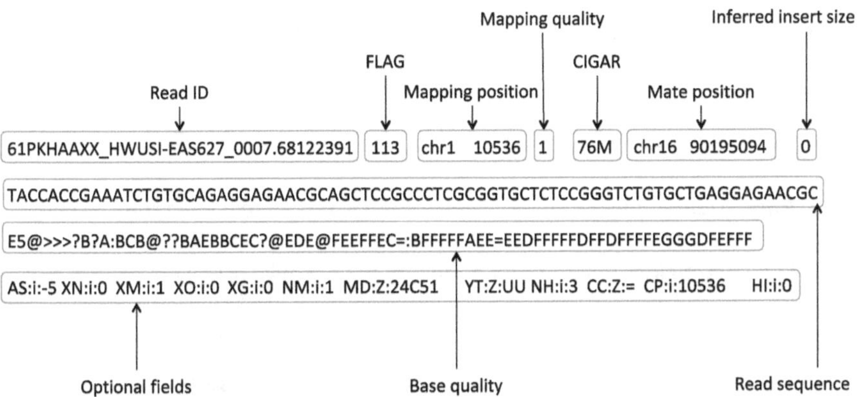

Figure 1.4: Alignment section example of the SAM format specification.

- **Read Id**: Unique identifier of the read. Corresponds to the *@SEQUENCE_ID* from the previous *fastq* example.

- **Flag**: Combination of bitwise flags indicating different properties of the alignment. For instance, 113 means the read is the first of a pair and it has been paired in the reverse strand. See for a detailed meaning of the flags.

- **Mapping position**: Chromosome and 1-based leftmost mapping position of the read in the reference genome.

- **Mapping quality**: Probability that the mapping is wrong. It equals to `-10log10P{mapping_position_is_wrong}` rounded to the nearest integer.

- **CIGAR**: String indicating the number of bases matching, mismatching, skipped, containing deletions or insertions with respect to the reference.

- **Mate position**: In paired-end data, the position where the pair of a read is mapped.

- **Inferred insert size**: In paired-end data, the inferred size of the insert between pair reads.

- **Read sequence**: Sequence of the read (second row from the *fastq* file).

- **Base quality**: Base quality of the sequence (fourth row from the *fastq* file).

- **Optional fields**: A list of predefined optional fields, usually extended by the aligners.

It is advisable to perform quality control of the mapped reads afterwards. This process allows the detection of random errors or other systematic biases that could not be discovered otherwise. The usage of graphical tools such as Qualimap [9] or command line tools such as SAMStat [10] makes this process straightforward by generating a very easy-to-interpret report.

1.2.3 Mapping post-processing

Almost every NGS analysis pipeline follows the steps described above. However, the post-processing step of the mapped data is particular for each sequencing technology (Figure 1.2). The aim of RNA-sequencing (RNA-Seq) experiments is the discovery of differentially expressed genes under certain conditions. Therefore, the step that follows the mapping process is the gene quantification. Quantifying the expression of a gene normally involves the estimation of the total number of reads mapped to each genic region, generating a text file containing the number of counts per gene. DNA-Seq analyses are focused on the detection of variants compared to a reference genome. These changes are mostly single-nucleotide polymorphisms (SNPs), but can also be small insertions or deletions, that accumulate as a result of evolution and, in a limited number of cases, can contribute or be the sole cause of a particular phenotype or disease. The process to obtain those variants is called *Variant calling*. As a result, a VCF file containing the genomic position of each variant as well as the alternative base or bases to the reference DNA will be generated. ChIP-Seq experiments measure how proteins interact with DNA to regulate gene expression, whereas DNase-Seq experiments identify the location of DNase I hypersensitive regions. In both cases, reads will normally concentrate on the mentioned areas in the form of peaks. In these cases, *peak calling* would be the following step. These results are reported in a basic BED file, a text tabular format containing the chromosome name, start and end positions and some optional descriptive features of the target areas. Methyl-Seq experiments aim to discover methylated pattern regions in the DNA that would significantly alter gene expression and chromatin remodelling. As in ChIP-Seq and DNase-Seq, methylated areas will also be reported in a BED file.

As indicated above, it is extremely important to measure the different sequencing errors or biases present in the data prior to analysis. In Chapter 3, many of these biases that can especially arise when trying to analyse data coming from different laboratories, sequencers or even when using replicates in RNA-Seq data analysis, will be addressed.

1.3 Applications of NGS

NGS technologies have a wide variety of applications. For instance, they have simplified the way to make *de novo* sequencing to reconstruct new genomes or transcriptomes from scratch, giving new insights into the biology of any organism, measuring how DNA or RNA sequences interact with proteins (ChIP-Seq[11] or CLIP-Seq[12]), or even study methylation patterns in genome-wide analysis

(Methyl-Seq) among others. Our laboratory focuses on the applications regarding transcriptome sequencing. This includes the discovery and analysis of both coding mRNA and non-coding RNA.

1.3.1 Functional characterisation of novel genes

There are two basic types of RNA: messenger RNAs (mRNAs), which are translated into proteins, and non-coding RNAs (ncRNAs), which are not. Despite the thought that only a small portion of the genome was functional (coding mRNAs), NGS technologies have revealed that nearly 90% of the human genome is actively transcribed in the form of non-coding RNAs [13, 14, 15]. These can be found in intronic and intergenic regions, and also antisense to some protein-coding genes. The vast majority of these new transcripts are non-coding and, despite earlier beliefs, there is growing evidence of their functional roles [16].

Non-coding RNAs can be basically grouped into two main groups depending on the transcript length: small non-coding RNAs (small ncRNAs) or long non-coding RNAs (lncRNAs). There are different types of small ncRNAs, such as transfer RNAs (tRNAs), which are carriers of the amino acids needed for the translation of mRNAs into proteins; micro RNAs (miRNAs), non-coding RNAs of approximately 22 nucleotides long that act in RNA silencing and post-transcriptional regulation of gene expression; ribosomal RNAs (rRNAs), which are the major structural components of the ribosome, essential for the protein synthesis; small nucleolar RNAs (snoRNAs), one of the most abundant classes of ncRNAs involved in the processing and modification of rRNAs, etc.

1.3.2   Long non-coding RNAs (lncRNAs)

Despite lncRNAs being the most abundant type of non-coding RNAs in the genome, they are still not well characterised. LncRNAs are generally defined as non-coding transcripts longer than 200 nucleotides [17, 18, 19, 20], known for being tissue-specific and important gene regulators. That regulation can be performed through different mechanisms [21]. For instance, lncRNAs can act as scaffolds that capture other molecules to target histone-modifying complexes to either activate or repress the expression of other genes [22]. LncRNAs generated from Alu SINE elements[1] can inhibit the transcription of specific mRNAs by binding to the RNA polymerase II as a cellular heat shock response [23]. They can also affect the formation of the transcription pre-initiation complex by creating a lncRNA-DNA triplex structure [24], as well as act as miRNA sponges by sequestering them and therefore, over-expressing genes that should have been repressed otherwise [25, 26, 27, 28], etc.

Most of the research is now focused on this area where the discovery and better characterisation of lncRNAs have gained in importance. Chapter 5 presents a new approach for the characterisation of lncRNAs integrating data from multiple and diverse tissues and cell lines. Furthermore, a new web prediction tool to detect lncRNAs acting as putative miRNA sponges, spongeScan, is also described.

1.3.3   Integrative analysis

Each omic technology has multiple applications. However, the combination of some of these technologies even increases their applicability. For instance, the combination of gene expression RNA-Seq with transcription factor (TF) ChIP-Seq or chromatin accessibility (DNase-Seq) permits the discrimination of direct from

---

[1]Primate-specific repeats comprising 11% of the human genome.

indirect targets of TFs [29] or the inference of transcriptional regulatory networks [30, 31]. Combining DNA methylation with RNA-Seq helps to identify global relationships between epigenetic changes and transcription [32, 33]. The integration of metabolomics and transcriptomics is useful to reveal the transcriptional control of metabolic fluxes [34], while the joint analysis of proteomics and RNA-Seq data is useful for the discovery of post-transcriptional control of protein levels [35].

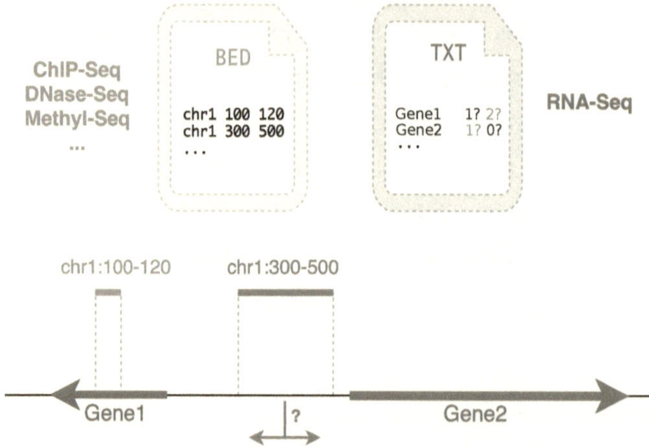

Figure 1.5: RNA-Seq analysis can benefit from the data integration of other omics such as ChIP-Seq, Methyl-Seq, etc. Special algorithms are needed to assign each regulatory region to the corresponding annotated genes. For regions such as the one in red might be unclear which gene it should be associated to.

However, while the statistical approaches followed to perform multi-omic analyses are essential to extract the most relevant information from the data, the algorithms needed to associate different types of data become equally important. For instance, all the application examples described above require connecting all positions where a transcription factor binds or a methylated motif to a region of a gene. This correspondence is normally performed based on its proximity to genes or transcripts (Figure 1.5) although it might be based on different criteria. Besides, there may be special conditions that require to be carefully managed to perform a proper connection. In Chapter 4, different algorithms publicly available are discussed and a new tool, RGmatch, is presented, which can be fully customised to cover all possible researcher needs.

Chapter 2

Motivation, aims and main contributions

2.1 Motivation

One of the most popular techniques used in computational biology is transcriptomics. Transcriptomics aims to describe the set of expressed transcripts and their regulation in different tissues, developmental stages or environmental conditions. Typically, in a quantitative transcriptomic experiment that studies transcriptional changes, samples at different conditions are sequenced to measure the gene expression and algorithms to identify gene expression differences are applied.

At the beginning of this PhD work, RNA-seq technology was starting to become a popular method to study gene expression. We participated in the SEQC project, an FDA initiative to study the quality of the different RNA-seq technologies available at that moment. That evaluation required the development of scripts and methods to assess the characteristics of RNA-seq platforms, screen a large number of samples, and compare technologies. Moreover, established bioinformatics tools to evaluate the quality of quantified RNA-seq data were not yet available. In Chapter 3 we describe our contribution to the SEQC project performing a comparative evaluation of RNA-seq technologies, and the development of the NOIseq package, one of the first R packages in providing a set of functions to systematically evaluate and normalise count data.

Once different sequencing technologies were established, there was an increasing interest in combining them to perform multiomics studies. STATegra is a FP7 project led by our group where several omics data types were generated for the same set of samples: RNA-seq, MicroRNA sequencing (miRNA-seq), Reduced-representation bisulfite sequencing (RRBS-Seq), DNase I hypersensitive sites sequencing (DNase-seq), Proteomics and Metabolomics. Some of these omics generate a BED file containing the regions of the genome where different genomics events happen. One first step to study the potential regulatory function of these events is to assign these regions to genes. No tools were available at that moment to associate BED regions to gene annotations in a flexible manner. In Chapter 4, I address the development of a Python tool to help in linking of genome regions to neighbouring genes.

One of the most exciting discoveries brought by the NGS technologies was the realisation that the human genome is not a large, repetitive and functionless nucleic acid sequence with just a small fraction of coding sequences, but that most of it is actively transcribed. Most of these new transcriptional players are non-coding and there was growing evidence of the functional effects of this extense battery of novel transcripts [17]. LncRNAs are a less characterised class of transcripts compared to small ncRNAs and since the beginning it was observed that they play an important role in gene regulation through different mechanisms. The last part of my book (Chapter 5) is motivated by these findings. We aimed to develop a *guilt-by-association* approach to functionally annotate lncRNAs as well as a web prediction resource to cover one of the regulation mechanisms lncRNAs might be involved in.

2.2   Specific aims

1. **To study the reproducibility and replicability of RNA-Seq by:**

   - Studying relevant biases that might affect any RNA-Seq analysis.

   - Assessing the robustness of this technology in terms of the number of replicates and sequencing depth .

2. **To create an R package to perform exploratory and differential expression analyses**

   Migrate the NOISeq algorithm into an R package following the Bioconductor guidelines and develop new exploratory tools.

3. **To create a tool to match genomic regions to features (genes, transcripts or exons)**

   There are some tools that are able to perform this task. However, none of them meets all the features we consider relevant for this purpose. As so, we will focus on creating a tool that:

- is easy to add in any analysis pipeline;

- is easily customised to report associations at any possible resolution (gene, transcript or exon);

- reports the annotated area of the gene involved;

- allows users to customise how these associations should be made (specify a maximum distance to a gene, prioritise different areas of a gene over others...);

- works for all the species;

- reports the distance to the associated feature;

- reports all overlapping genes.

4. **Create a methodology to functionally characterise lncRNAs**

The functions of a small fraction of lncRNAs have been already studied in depth. We aim at creating a new methodology to functionally characterise lncRNAs to better understand the processes in which they might be involved. To do so, we will:

- download and use public data from different tissues and cell lines;

- use a *guilt-by-association* approach to annotate lncRNAs with the functions of the protein-coding genes they might correlate with.

5. **Develop a new tool to predict miRNA binding elements in lncRNA sequences**

One of the mechanisms by which lncRNAs might act as regulators is by sequestering miRNAs. In this particular case, we will focus on:

- creating an algorithm to predict these miRNA sequestration events;

- developing a new web tool to easily calculate and visualise these predictions in a user-friendly way.

2.3   Main contributions

2.3.1   *Journal papers*

1. SEQC/MAQC-III Consortium.
   A Comprehensive Assessment of RNA-Seq Accuracy, Reproducibility and Information Content by the Sequencing Quality Control Consortium.
   Nature Biotechnology 32 (9): 903-14. **2014 Sep**
   388 cites when checked on the 2nd of March 2020.

2. Tarazona S, Furió-Tarí P, Turrà D, Pietro AD, Nueda MJ, Ferrer A, Conesa A.
   Data Quality Aware Analysis of Differential Expression in RNA-Seq with NOISeq R/Bioc Package.
   Nucleic Acids Research 43 (21). **2015 Dec**
   142 cites when checked on the 2nd of March 2020.

3. Furió-Tarí P, Tarazona S, Gabaldón T, Enright AJ, Conesa A.
   spongeScan: A web for detecting microRNA binding elements in lncRNA sequences.
   Nucleic Acids Res. 44(W1):W176-80. doi: 10.1093/nar/gkw443. Epub 2016 May 19. **2016 Jul**
   24 cites and **115** accesses a month on average when checked on the 2nd of March 2020.

4. De Panis DN, Padró J, <u>Furió-Tarí P</u>, Tarazona S, Milla Carmona PS, Soto IM, Dopazo H, Conesa A, Hasson E.
Transcriptome modulation during host shift is driven by secondary metabolites in desert Drosophila.
Mol Ecol. 25(18):4534-50. doi: 10.1111/mec.13785. Epub 2016 Sep 6. **2016 Sep**
17 cites when checked on the 2nd of March 2020.

5. <u>Furió-Tarí P</u>, Conesa A, Tarazona S.
RGmatch: matching genomic regions to proximal genes in omics data integration.
BMC Bioinformatics. 17(Suppl 15):427. doi: 10.1186/s12859-016-1293-1. **2016 Nov**
3 cites when checked on the 2nd of March 2020.

6. García-Molinero V, García-Martínez J, Reja R, <u>Furió-Tarí P</u>, Antúnez O, Vinay-achandran V, Conesa A, Pugh BF, Pérez-Ortín JE, Rodríguez-Navarro S.
The SAGA/TREX-2 subunit Sus1 binds widely to transcribed genes and affects mRNA turnover globally.
Epigenetics Chromatin. 11(1):13. doi: 10.1186/s13072-018-0184-2. **2018 Mar**
3 cites when checked on the 2nd of March 2020.

7. Hernández-de-Diego R, Tarazona S, Martínez-Mira C, Balzano-Nogueira L, <u>Furió-Tarí P</u>, Pappas GJ Jr, Conesa A.
PaintOmics 3: a web resource for the pathway analysis and visualization of multi-omics data.
Nucleic Acids Res. 46(W1):W503-W509. doi: 10.1093/nar/gky466 **2018 Jul**
12 cites when checked on the 2nd of March 2020.

2.3.2 Conferences

- *HiTSeq 2013* Berlin, Germany. July, 2013. Tarazona S, <u>Furió-Tarí Pedro</u>, Turrà D, Di Pietro A, Ferrer A, and Conesa A. Quality-control, experimental design and FDR controlled differential expression of RNA-seq with the NOISeq R package.

- *Congreso Argentino de Bioinformática y Biología Computacional* Rosario, Argentina. October, 2013. De Panis, D, <u>Furió-Tarí P</u>, Padró J, Tarazona S, Dopazo H, Conesa A, Hasson E. Transcriptomics of host adaption, early results: Gene expression patterns of the cactophilic fly *Drosophila buzzatii* in its natural breeding and feeding resources.

- *SMODIA 2015* Valencia, Spain. September 2015. <u>Furió-Tarí P</u>, Tarazona S, Conesa A. RGmatch: Matching genomic regions to proximal genes in omics data integration.

- *SMODIA 2015* Valencia, Spain. September 2015. Hernández-De-Diego R, <u>Furió-Tarí P</u>, Tarazona S, Conesa A. Paintomics 3.0: Integrated visualization of multi omics data on KEGG pathways.

- *JBI 2016 - XIII Symposium on Bioinformatics* Valencia, Spain. May, 2016. Tarazona S, <u>Furió-Tarí P</u>, Turrà D, Di Pietro A, Nueda MJ, Ferrer A, Conesa A. Data quality aware analysis of differential expression in RNA-seq with NOISeq R/Bioc package.

- *JBI 2016 - XIII Symposium on Bioinformatics* Valencia, Spain. May, 2016. Hernández-De-Diego R, <u>Furió-Tarí P</u>, Tarazona S, Conesa A. Integrative visualization of multi-omics data: The PaintOmics 3 platform.

- *JBI 2016 - XIII Symposium on Bioinformatics* Valencia, Spain. May, 2016. Tarazona S, Martínez C, <u>Furió-Tarí P</u>, Gómez D, Conesa A. Tools for the design and analysis of multi-omic experiments.

- *RegGen SIG 2017* Prague, Czech Republic. July 2017. Hernández-De-Diego R, <u>Furió-Tarí P</u>, Tarazona S, Conesa A. Integrative visualization of multi-omics data: The PaintOmics 3 platform.

- *RegGen SIG 2017* Prague, Czech Republic. July 2017. Tarazona S, Clemente M, Hernández-De-Diego R, Gómez D, <u>Furió-Tarí P</u>, Martínez C, Conesa A. The challenge of integrating multi-omic multi-factorial data to infer regulatory networks.

- *JBI 2018 - XIV Symposium on Bioinformatics* Granada, Spain. November, 2018. Hernández-de-Diego R, Tarazona S, Martínez-Mira C, Balzano-Nogueira L, <u>Furió-Tarí P</u>, Pappas G, Conesa A. PaintOmics 3: a web resource for the pathway analysis and visualization of multi-omics data.

2.3.3 Software

- <u>Furió-Tarí P</u>, Conesa A, Tarazona S.
  RGmatch, Python tool.

- <u>Furió-Tarí P</u>, Tarazona S, Gabaldón T, Enright AJ, Conesa A.
  SpongeScan, web resource.

- Tarazona S, <u>Furió-Tarí P</u>, Turrà D, Pietro AD, Nueda MJ, Ferrer A, Conesa A
  NOISeq, Bioconductor R package.

Hernández-de-Diego R, Tarazona S, Martínez-Mira C, Balzano-Nogueira L,
<u>Furió-Tarí P</u>, Pappas GJ Jr, Conesa A.
PaintOmics 3, web resource.

2.3.4 Courses

I have been teaching to the scientific community in these courses:

- International Course of Massive Data Analysis (Centro de Investigación Príncipe Felipe, Valencia). Year 2013 and 2014 in IX and X editions. Lectures about the RNA-Seq pipeline analysis (Quality control, mapping, counting...).

- The Genomics of Gene Expression RNA-Seq course (Centro de Investigación Príncipe Felipe, Valencia). Year 2014 and 2015 in 1st and 2nd edition. Lectures about the RNA-Seq pipeline analysis (Quality control, mapping, counting...).

2.3.5 Scientific visits

Fellowship at the *Functional genomics and analysis of small RNA function group* (Dr. Anton Enright group), The European Bioinformatics Institute (EMBL-EBI) in Hinxton, UK.
April - June 2014
Development of a miRNA sponge prediction tool in lncRNAs

Scientific visit at the *Computational Biology Lab - High Performance Computing Service* (Ignacio Medina group), University of Cambridge, UK.

August - October 2015

Development of a web tool for massive NGS analysis

Fellowship at the *Department of Molecular Genetics and Microbiology, Genetics Institute* (Dr. Lauren McIntyre group), University of Florida, Gainesville (USA).

November - December 2015

Development of a miRNA sponge prediction tool in lncRNAs

Chapter 3

Quality Analysis of RNA-Seq technology

The work performed of this chapter led to the following publications:

SEQC/MAQC-III Consortium.

A Comprehensive Assessment of RNA-Seq Accuracy, Reproducibility and Information Content by the Sequencing Quality Control Consortium.

Nature Biotechnology 32 (9): 903-14. **2014**

Tarazona, Sonia, Pedro Furió-Tarí, David Turrà, Antonio Di Pietro, María José Nueda, Alberto Ferrer, and Ana Conesa.

Data Quality Aware Analysis of Differential Expression in RNA-Seq with NOISeq R/Bioc Package.

Nucleic Acids Research 43 (21). **2015**

3.1   Introduction

The transcriptome is the complete set of transcripts in a cell, as well as their abundance for a specific developmental stage or physiological condition. Understanding the transcriptome is vital to functionally characterize the elements of which it is composed and so, understand development and disease.

RNA sequencing (RNA-Seq) is an approach based on high-throughput sequencing for both mapping and quantifying transcriptomes with many advantages over other existing approaches [36]. The first one is the ability to sequence genome-wide, making it attractive for non-model organisms in which genomic sequences are yet unknown. Secondly, it is suitable to study complex transcriptomes because the reads reveal the connectivity between exons at single-nucleotide resolution. Moreover, this technology is more sensitive for genes expressed at high or low levels, having a much bigger dynamic range than other approaches depending on the sequencing depth.

However, different aspects must be checked and considered beforehand to assess the reliability of the results obtained during the analysis. For example, it is really important to evaluate the quality of the samples sequenced, whether there were any artefacts introduced by the sequencing process or not, the sequencing depth (total number of reads present in the file), read length, etc. Another important aspect, unknown at the time this research was done, was the study of replicability of the technology.

Many of the RNA-Seq analyses are made using the object-oriented programming language called R [37], as they require some powerful statistical computation. R is a free software environment for statistical computing and graphics. It compiles and runs on almost all the recent UNIX, Windows and MacOS platforms. One of the most important characteristics of R is its easiness of use and the ability to import other packages containing the tools to address specific analyses. The most important R package repository for the analysis and comprehension of high-throughput genomic data is Bioconductor [38, 39], which is open source.

At the time of this research, there was no freely available software to study the most important quality parameters of an RNA-Seq experiment. One of the contributions made to this chapter is the development of a Bioconductor package that could be used by the scientific community to assess the quality of the samples sequenced in RNA-Seq experiments including an already existing differentially expression algorithm developed in our group called NOISeq.

Another aspect not previously evaluated, was the study of the reproducibility of next-generation sequencing platforms such as RNA-Seq. In this chapter, we also present our contribution to the SEQC project studying this feature. The SEQC project is a continuation of the MAQC project, an initiative that the FDA began in 2005 to evaluate the reproducibility of microarray platforms.

3.2　Objectives

- Creation of a Bioconductor package for the quality assessment of RNA-Seq data.

- Evaluation of the reproducibility and replicability of RNA-Seq technology as part of the SEQC project.

3.3   NOISeq

Despite all the advantages of RNA-Seq technology, sequencing artefacts present in the final datasets could potentially lead to biased and misleading conclusions in the analysis. Therefore, early detection of these biases is of huge importance to correct or discard noisy datasets. Apart from the ability to run differential expression analysis, NOISeq provides the necessary tools to assess the quality control of the samples, allowing to check for the possible biases that could be present in the samples and the tools to correct and normalise these data.

NOISeq is an open access R package, currently published in Bioconductor. R is an object oriented programming (OOP) language containing classes, methods and attributes.

The NOISeq algorithm was mainly developed by Dr Tarazona and was part of her PhD book [40]. The NOISeq statistical method and the biological meaning of the quality control tools can be found explained in detail there. My contribution to this package was the design of a logical workflow and the development of proper data models that make it more user-friendly and would suit Bioconductor requirements.

3.3.0.1   *The package*

NOISeq contains a set of tools to perform the three following different tasks represented in Figure 3.1:

- quality control of the samples by doing different exploratory plots;

- normalisation and filtering of the data by applying different statistical methods;

- differential expression analysis.

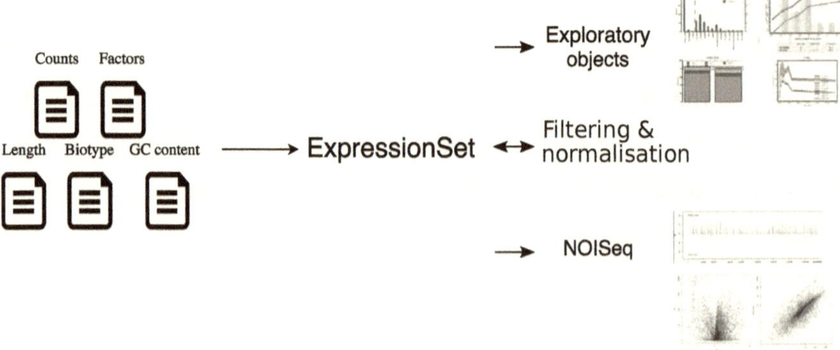

Figure 3.1: Outline of NOISeq package functionalities.

Base R provides different OOP systems: S3 and S4. S4 classes represent a more formal and rigorous design compared to S3. This is because S3 classes lack any validation, allowing any object to be easily converted to an S3 object by running one single line even if the original object has nothing to do with this type of class. However, S4 objects have to be specifically created using the constructor function, so programmers can write code to validate the parameters supplied to create the new object, preventing possible errors. For these reasons, different S4 classes (Figure 3.2) were implemented to store the relevant information needed to perform each of these tasks.

In order to work with NOISeq, the user needs to have at least a matrix of counts with one row per gene or transcript and one column per condition and a matrix of factors used to perform the differential expression analysis. Additionally, users can also provide a matrix of genomic positions used to perform *Manhattan* plots where the expression of up and down regulated genes is highlighted across chromosomal positions, an array of biotypes to perform other meaningful exploratory

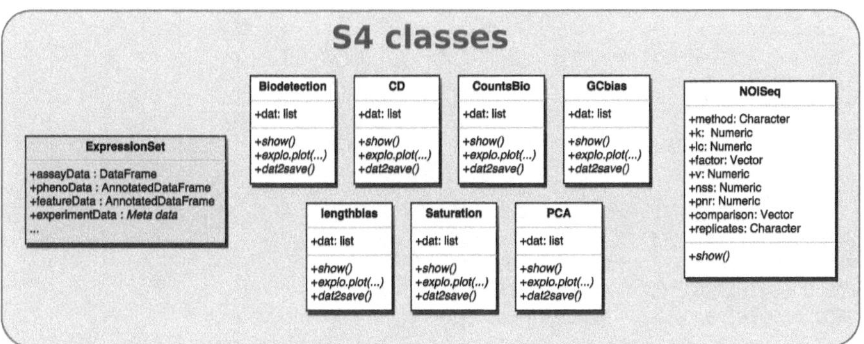

Figure 3.2: S4 classes used in NOISeq package.

plots per biotype as well as an array containing the lengths of the genes or transcripts introduced in the matrix of counts to be able to apply normalisation methods. All this information will be incorporated in NOISeq using one of the methods called *readData* as can be seen in the example below.

```
# Install Bioconductor repository manager
> if (!requireNamespace("BiocManager", quietly = TRUE))
+     install.packages("BiocManager")

# Install NOISeq
> BiocManager::install("NOISeq")

# Load NOISeq
> library(NOISeq)

# Load default example NOISeq dataset
> data(Marioni)

# Explore data from the dataset
> head(mycounts)
                R1L1Kidney R1L2Liver R1L3Kidney R1L4Liver R1L6Liver R1L7Kidney
ENSG00000177757          2         1          0         0         1          2
ENSG00000187634         49        27         43        34        23         41
ENSG00000188976         73        34         77        56        45         68
ENSG00000187961         15         8         15        13        11         13
```

```
> head(myfactors)
          Tissue TissueRun
R1L1Kidney Kidney  Kidney_1
R1L2Liver  Liver   Liver_1
R1L3Kidney Kidney  Kidney_1

> head(mychroms)
                Chr GeneStart GeneEnd
ENSG00000177757  1     742614  745077
ENSG00000187634  1     850393  869824
ENSG00000188976  1     869459  884494
ENSG00000187961  1     885830  890958

> head(mybiotypes)
  ENSG00000177757   ENSG00000187634   ENSG00000188976   ENSG00000187961
       "lincRNA" "protein_coding" "protein_coding" "protein_coding"

> head(mylength)
ENSG00000177757 ENSG00000187634 ENSG00000188976 ENSG00000187961
         2464.0          4985.0          3870.5          4964.0

# Load dataset data into main ExpressionSet S4 class
> mydata <- readData(data=mycounts, biotype=mybiotypes, chromosome=mychroms,
                                 factors=myfactors, length = mylength)
```

In order to store all this information, the S4 *ExpressionSet* object was used [39]. This object was originally created to load and manipulate microarray data in R, but it can be also used to store NGS data for the same purposes. As so, this object contains different slots, which are prepared to store all the relevant information. NOISeq uses three of these slots: *assayData* to store the expression data from NGS experiments (counts), *phenoData* to store the 'metadata' describing the samples in the experiment (factors) and *featureData* to store the annotations and metadata about the features introduced (length, GC content, chromosome information and/or biotypes). Below there is an example of the *ExpressionSet* object with the three slots used by NOISeq underlined.

```
> mydata
```

```
ExpressionSet (storageMode: lockedEnvironment)
assayData: 5088 features, 10 samples
  element names: exprs
protocolData: none
phenoData
  sampleNames: R1L1Kidney R1L2Liver ... R2L6Kidney (10 total)
  varLabels: Tissue TissueRun
  varMetadata: labelDescription
featureData
  featureNames: ENSG00000177757 ENSG00000187634 ... ENSG00000201145 (5088 total)
  fvarLabels: Length Biotype ... GeneEnd (5 total)
  fvarMetadata: labelDescription
experimentData: use 'experimentData(object)'
Annotation:
```

The normalisation and filtering of data takes the *ExpressionSet* object as the main input and returns a new object of the same class with transformed data.

The *ExpressionSet* object will also be taken as input for the 10 diagnostic and visualisation plots available in the package. However, this object is used as an intermediate object only. Each of the plots requires a different transformation of the main data, which is performed by calling to the *dat()* function. This function takes as an additional parameter the plot type and, depending on the choice, the data will be transformed and filtered accordingly. The type of plots accepted will be one of *biodetection, cd, countsbio, GCbias, lengthbias, saturation* or *PCA* [40], corresponding to the ones in Figure 3.2. Taking advantage of S4 classes available in R [37], different classes were defined for the different plots. This way, the researcher is able to use the same functions independently of the plot to be performed. When calling the *dat()* function and specifying the plot of choice as an argument, the function will return the corresponding class object. *show()*, which prints a nice summary of the object, *explo.plot()*, which plots the desired figure, and *dat2save()*, which returns an object containing the most relevant information regarding the plot to be stored, methods have been implemented for the 7 S4 classes. This is useful from the user perspective as these methods will always work with any of those objects without the user having to deal with different functions.

The plots are performed in 2 steps because of the following reasons:

- transforming the *ExpressionSet* object sometimes requires a few seconds and the transformed object can be used multiple times to generate plots that are made instantly based on some additional parameters/filters;

- the transformed object can be stored in a binary object after applying the method *dat2save()* implemented for the 7 S4 classes. This method will transform each of the objects into a more user-friendly R object containing the most relevant information.

Finally, once the researcher is confident with the quality of the data, it is possible to apply the *noiseq()* function to perform the differential expression analysis step. The two approaches, NOISeq, for technical replicates or no replicates, and NOISeqBio, for biological replicates, take the same *ExpressionSet* object as input, but a different type of object was needed to store NOISeq results. As mentioned above, all the NOISeq parameters are stored in different slots, as well as the results obtained by the algorithm, which are stored in a *data.frame.* The *NOISeq* output class also has the *show()* method implemented that allows the researcher to see a summary of the content of the output object. Furthermore, a *degenes()* function was also developed that uses the *NOISeq* S4 output object to easily gather the differentially expressed genes on one or both conditions depending on the probability threshold introduced. Below there is an example of how to calculate differentially expressed genes using the NOISeq function.

```
> mynoiseq = noiseq(mydata, k = 0.5, norm = "rpkm", replicates = "technical",
                factor="Tissue", pnr = 0.2, nss = 5, v = 0.02, lc = 1)
```

```
[1] "Computing (M,D) values..."
[1] "Computing probability of differential expression..."

> mynoiseq

You are comparing Kidney - Liver from Tissue

                Kidney_mean Liver_mean          M          D prob     ranking
ENSG00000163399  1289.54326    41.57492  4.955003 1247.9683    1   1247.9782
ENSG00000132703    91.67521  5083.56952 -5.793166 4991.8943    1  -4991.8977
ENSG00000132693    44.67117  4058.28607 -6.505383 4013.6149    1  -4013.6202
ENSG00000158874    89.12252  7626.56264 -6.419099 7537.4401    1  -7537.4429
ENSG00000172482    11.80019   925.76684 -6.293767  913.9667    1   -913.9883
ENSG00000055957    14.52202  1092.84712 -6.233706 1078.3251    1  -1078.3431
                Length Chrom GeneStart    GeneEnd        Biotype
ENSG00000163399 12876.0     1 116717359 116748917 protein_coding
ENSG00000132703  1041.0     1 157824240 157825284 protein_coding
ENSG00000132693  2056.5     1 157948704 157951003 protein_coding
ENSG00000158874  1311.0     1 159458707 159460042 protein_coding
ENSG00000172482  4724.0     2 241456835 241467210 protein_coding
ENSG00000055957  3163.0     3  52786648  52801117 protein_coding

Normalisation
        method: rpkm
        k: 0.5
        lc: 1

You are working with technical replicates
```

3.3.0.2   The functions

As explained in the above section, different S4 classes were implemented to perform the exploratory plots. Considering the *ExpressionSet* as the main input and the plot as the final output, the whole process could last from a couple of seconds to half a minute depending on the chosen exploratory plot. Many times, the result obtained the first time might not be as desired (maybe the user wants a bigger font size, different range limits, even plotting a different sample...), but the flexibility of the function allows the user to tweak the options until the expected plot is obtained.

The most time-consuming process in the algorithm is the transformation of the relevant data from the *ExpressionSet* to a format that is easy to work with in order to plot according to other user's parameters. For this reason, the two-step approach mentioned above was implemented to compute the different exploratory plots. Firstly, data is transformed to the needed format depending on the exploratory plot to be displayed and, secondly, this transformed data is used as the input for the plotting function. This way, the user can re-run the plot from the transformed data multiple times in a second. A simple change of parameters will be required to improve the graphical display.

To simplify the usage of different methods to calculate each plot, an object-oriented S4 system approach was used. For example, to do the Biodetection plot, users need to first call *biodetection.dat()* followed by *biodetection.plot()*, or *cd.dat()* and *cd.plot()* respectively to make a CD plot. For this reason, a generic *dat()* function was implemented. Depending on the main parameter given (a string containing one of *biodetection, cd, countsbio, GCbias , lengthbias, saturation* or *PCA*), this method internally calls one of *biodetection.dat(), cd.dat(), countsbio.dat(), GCbias.dat(), lengthbias.dat(), saturation.dat()*, or *PCA.dat()* respectively, and return an instance of the corresponding S4 class. Generic *show(), dat2save()* and *explo.plot()* methods were created to manipulate the transformed data. The different S4 classes override these three methods and implement them differently. Users will need to know only two methods, which are *dat()* and *explo.plot()*. The first one will return an instance of the S4 class depending on the plot of choice, and the second one will consume that object and automatically generate the requested plot.

An example of this implementation is shown below:

```
> mydata2plot = dat(mydata, type = "biodetection", k = 0)
[1] "Biotypes detection is to be computed for:"
 [1] "R1L1Kidney" "R1L2Liver"  "R1L3Kidney" "R1L4Liver"  "R1L6Liver"
```

```
[6] "R1L7Kidney" "R1L8Liver"  "R2L2Kidney""R2L3Liver"  "R2L6Kidney"

> explo.plot(mydata2plot, samples=1)
```

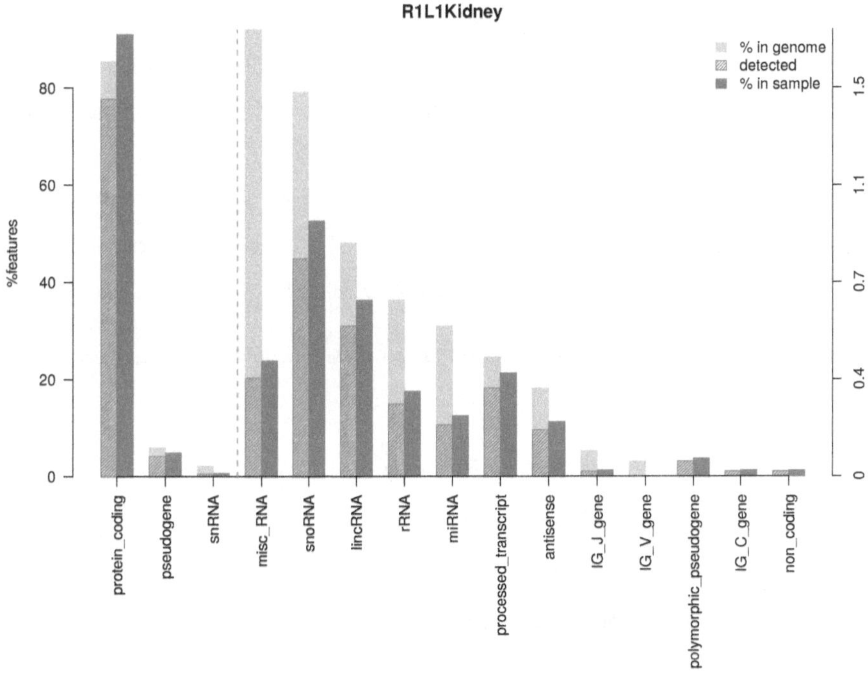

Figure 3.3: Biodetection plot from NOISeq.

3.4 Sequence Quality Control (SEQC) project

3.4.1 *Dataset*

The SEQC project, led by the Food and Drug Administration (FDA, United States) aimed to assess the reproducibility and replicability of RNA-Seq analyses. In this study, six different samples (A-F) were sequenced. Samples A and B contained Universal Human Reference RNA (UHRR) and Human Brain Reference RNA (HBRR), respectively, plus spike-ins of synthetic RNA from the External RNA Control Consortium (ERCC). Samples A and B were mixed in known ratios, 3:1 and 1:3, to construct samples C and D, respectively. Spike-ins were also sequenced separately to assess dynamic range (samples E and F). All the samples were distributed to several independent sites for RNA-Seq library construction and profiling by Illumina's Hiseq 2000 and Life Technologies' SOLiD 5500. Vendors created their own cDNA libraries, which were distributed to each test site to examine 'site effects' independent of the library preparation. A total of 108 libraries were sequenced on Hiseq 2000 for samples A to D and 68 on SOLiD.

Our analysis was focused on the Illumina samples. These were sequenced by six different laboratories:

- AGR: *Australian Genome Research Facility*

- BGI: *Beijing Genomics Institute*

- CNL: *Cognitive Neuroscience Laboratory (Cornell University)*

- COH: *Beckman Research Institute of City of Hope*

- MAY: *Mayo Clinic Florida*

- NVS: *Novartis*

Every library had a unique barcode sequence at each site, and was pooled before sequencing, so each lane was sequencing the same material, allowing a study of lane-specific effects. Besides, four replicate libraries were used for each sample A to D per site. In addition, a fifth replicate was also used by BGI, CNL and MAY laboratories. The samples followed the following name convention:

- Project (SEQC for all the libraries)

- Platform (ILM in our case)

- Site

- RNA Sample Type (A, B, C, D, E or F)

- Replicate Number

- Lane/Sector Number

- Index Barcode

- Flow-cell Barcode

- Read Direction (R1 or R2 for pair-end data)

The sequencing depth of samples A and B in all the laboratories can be found in Table 3.1. The numbers show the total number of reads per replicate (all reads from different lanes are added) and per laboratory.

Lab	Sequencing depth (million reads per replicate)											
	A1	A2	A3	A4	A5	Total A	B1	B2	B3	B4	B5	Total B
AGR	346	363	307	451	-	1467	361	394	356	334	-	1445
BGI	211	174	205	236	209	1035	235	232	245	181	137	1030
CNL	207	191	127	254	148	927	208	218	217	183	118	944
COH	212	214	213	208	-	847	198	203	201	193	-	795
MAY	137	264	196	448	116	1161	240	211	242	249	88	1030
NVS	345	400	370	378	-	1493	335	343	358	365	-	1401

Table 3.1: Sequencing depth of the samples per laboratory and replicate.

3.4.2 Methods

Raw reads contain not only the sequence but also the quality of each base, which represents the likelihood of the base having been properly called by the sequencer. FastQC [6] is a popular tool to analyse data quality and extract other relevant statistics such as the mean GC content, read length distribution, duplication levels, adapter content, etc. This tool was was used to get an overview of the quality of the data and the results were used as input to perform Principal Component Analyses (PCA) to check for biases. The reads were mapped using TopHat v1.4.1 [41] using *Homo Sapiens* GRCh37.66 as the reference genome. TopHat was chosen because it was the most widely used by the scientific community that could deal with splice events. Cufflinks v2.0.0 [19] was used to build new unannotated transcripts and quantify the expression of transcripts and genes in Fragments Per Kilobase Of Exon Per Million Fragments Mapped (FPKM). Finally, the NOISeq package [42, 40] was used to perform quality analysis of the data. All the analysis were performed developing either Bash, Python or R scripts.

3.4.3   Results

3.4.3.1   Quality control of raw data

First of all, the quality of all the different samples was checked separately using FastQC. Taking into account all the different laboratories, replicates and lanes per sample, a total of 3664 *fastq* files were managed. Taking advantage of the summary reports that FastQC generates for every analysis, a PCA was built. Basically, a 0, 1 or 2 was assigned to passed, warning and failed tests resulting in a final matrix of 3664 x 11 dimensions. Figure 3.4 shows the results of the QC. The PCA was coloured by laboratory (Figure 3.4a) showing a scattered plot that pointed to laboratory biasese. The most important factor that explained the 40% variance in the first component was the sequence quality per base. This same PCA was also coloured by sample (Figure 3.4b) showing a clear distinction between samples A-D and E-F (spike-in samples), as expected. This fact was explained by the second principal component, in which the most important factor was the GC content and the sequence duplication levels. Samples A to D were found grouped together suggesting that there was not a sample bias.

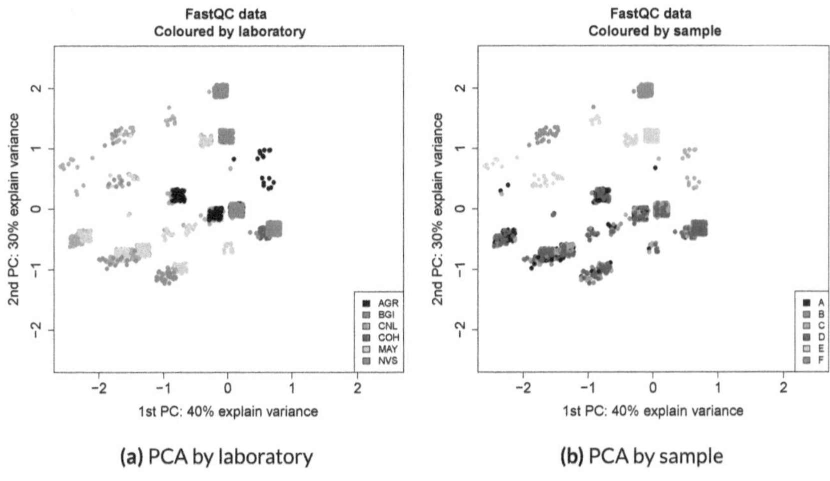

(a) PCA by laboratory   (b) PCA by sample

Figure 3.4: PCA analysis of FastQC output

The NOISeq package was used to extract relevant information to perform the quality analysis after mapping the reads. Parameters, such as saturation dynamics (number of genes detected according to the sequencing depth levels), new detection levels (number of new genes detected per additional million reads), biotype relative detection (percentage of biotypes detected in sample) and a summary of the number of reads per biotype (1st quartile, median and 3rd quartile) were extracted. All this data was used to build a big matrix with as many rows as the number of mapped samples and as many columns as the amount of information extracted from NOISeq. This matrix was used to build the PCA in Figure 3.5. As shown, there was an evident separation between the different samples. In fact, the first component, explaining 67.5% of the variance, was distinguishing between the *spike-in* samples (E-F) and the actual samples (A-D). This component was mainly influenced by the total number of reads mapping to pseudogenes, as well as the percentage of ribosomal RNA (rRNA) detected within the annotated human reference genome. The second component, which was actually separating the samples

A-D and explaining 6.5% of the variance, was influenced by the quartiles of rRNA content present in the mitochondria.

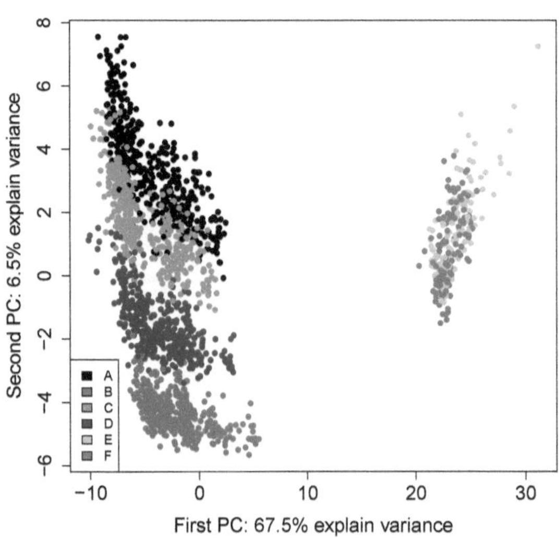

Figure 3.5: PCA of SEQC samples analysed by NOIseq read count quality parameters. Lanes and replicates are shown as different entities. Data are coloured by sample type.

3.4.3.2 *Quality analysis from mapped reads*

Due to the good separation between the samples and controls in Figure 3.5, samples E-F were filtered out and the PCA analysis re-run. The new PCA was coloured by sample (Figure 3.6) showing a clear separation of samples, with no bias detected. On the contrary, when the same PCA was coloured by laboratory (Figure 3.7), a clear separation was evident considering both components, indicating a laboratory associated bias in the data. Data appeared clustered into two groups. One group was composed by AGR, COH and NVS samples, and the second

contained BGI, CNL and MAY samples. Interestingly, the first group of laboratories had a greater sequencing depth than those of the second. Taking this into
account, the PCA was coloured again, but this time by sequencing depth using a
colour gradient (Figure 3.8), confirming that the separation made by the PCA was
due to the different sequencing depth obtained from the different laboratories.
This confirmed previous work from our laboratory where we showed that the sequencing depth is an important factor to be taken into account when analysing
RNA-Seq samples [42].

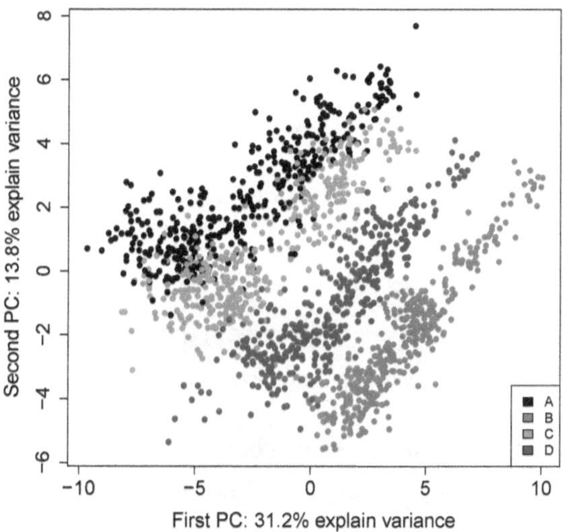

Figure 3.6: PCA of SEQC samples analysed by NOIseq read count quality parameters. Lanes
and replicates are shown as different entities. Data are coloured by sample type. Samples E & F
were excluded.

Besides analysing the biases, correlation analyses of the expression levels in FPKM
were also performed (Figure 3.9). The upper triangular matrix shows the correlation of gene expression levels and the lower triangular matrix the correlation of

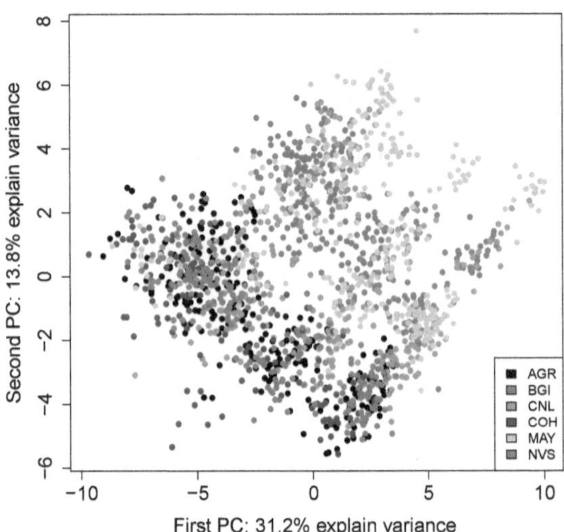

Figure 3.7: PCA of SEQC samples analysed by NOIseq read count quality parameters. Lanes and replicates are shown as different entities. Data are coloured by laboratory. Samples E & F were excluded.

transcript expression levels between replicates of the same laboratory for samples A and B (only sample B is shown in Figure 3.9 but results are comparable).

Results from Figure 3.9 showed a strong correlation between replicates. However, there was one laboratory, MAY, which correlated worst in general. In fact, replicate 5 of sample B had a correlation value of around 0.5. The replicate had the lowest sequencing depth, which could explain the differences in correlation. Therefore, this replicate was treated as an outlier and removed from further analyses.

After that, correlation between the mean expression levels obtained by the different laboratories was also performed (Figure 3.10).

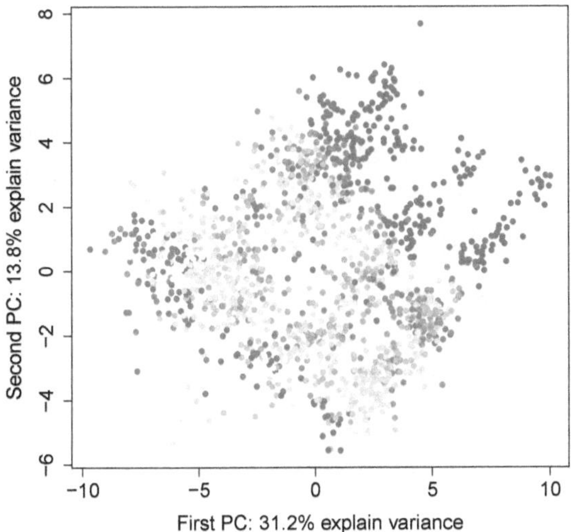

Figure 3.8: PCA of SEQC samples analysed by NOIseq read count quality parameters. Lanes and replicates are shown as different entities. Data are coloured by sequencing depth. Samples E & F were excluded. Yellow indicates higher sequencing depth than red colours.

The results obtained, shown in Figure 3.10, supported, even more, the importance of the sequencing depth. Samples with better correlation values were actually the ones with the highest sequencing depth levels. Therefore, although normalisation steps were applied, sequencing depth bias was still present, showing the strong impact it has on data analysis.

3.4.3.3   Differential expression analysis

One of the objectives of the current study was to evaluate the robustness of the analysis of differentially expressed genes between samples A and B as a function of the sequencing technology and laboratory, as well as detecting any associated

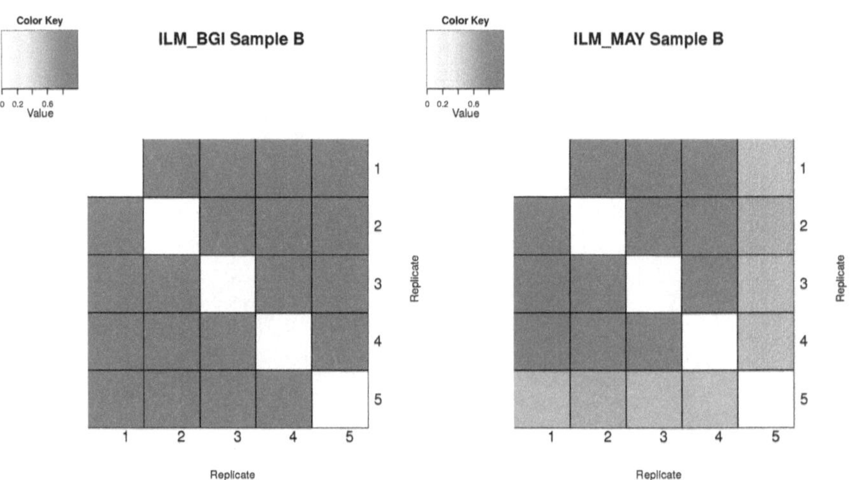

Figure 3.9: Correlation between replicates of sample B in two different laboratories. Upper triangular matrix shows gene correlations and lower triangular matrix shows transcript correlations.

biases. The NOISeq package, explained in section 3.3 was used for this purpose. Table 3.2 shows differentially expressed genes in common between laboratories. A larger amount of overexpressed genes was found in sample A over B. This could have a biological explanation because of the fact that sample A was composed by a mix of tissues, whereas sample B only contained brain tissue. Another conclusion that could be also extracted from the table, is that laboratories with higher sequencing depths detect more differentially expressed genes, highlighting, once again, the importance of the sequencing depth. For example, the higher number of overexpressed genes in sample A for the AGR laboratory (7950) compared to MAY (6097) can be explained by the sequencing depth differences. In fact, the percentage of commonly overexpressed genes detected in MAY that was also detected in AGR is 97% for sample A and 96.3% for sample B, indicating great robustness and reproducibility of the RNA-Seq technology.

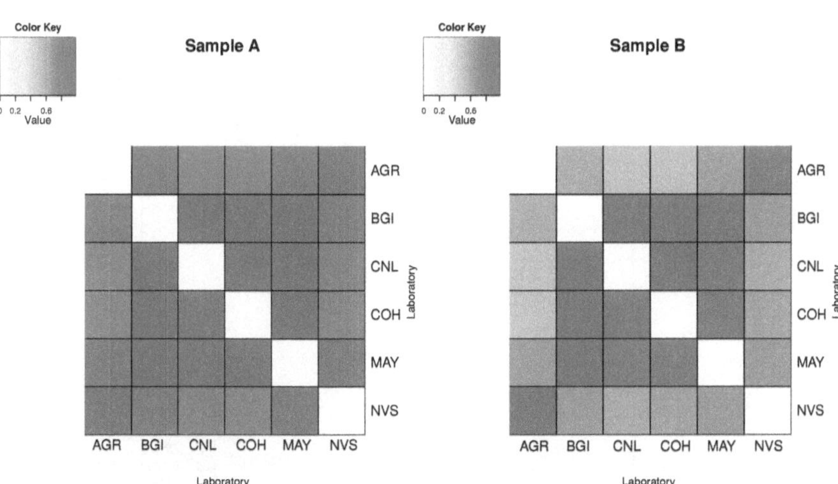

Figure 3.10: Correlation of gene expression values for the same samples run at different laboratories. Mean expression values across 4 replicates are used to calculate correlations between laboratories. Upper triangular matrix shows gene correlations and lower triangular matrix shows transcript correlations.

	AGR	BGI	CNL	COH	MAY	NVS	Total A
AGR	-	6228	5965	7240	5901	6984	**7950**
BGI	3929	-	5681	6115	5493	6167	**6330**
CNL	3892	3690	-	5923	5388	5902	**6188**
COH	4745	3906	3886	-	5902	6868	**7875**
MAY	4032	3653	3637	4046	-	5839	**6097**
NVS	4507	3899	3857	4473	3982	-	**7298**
Total B	**5070**	**4016**	**4026**	**5336**	**4187**	**4770**	

Table 3.2: Differentially expressed genes in common between laboratories for samples A (upper quadrant) & B (lower quadrant).

To study more in detail the sequencing depth effect, differential expression was measured again taking more lanes into account progressively. From 1 to 8 available lanes were selected randomly resampling 5 times.

Figure 3.11 showed that the amount of differentially expressed genes depended directly on the sequencing depth of the sample. The higher the sequencing depth,

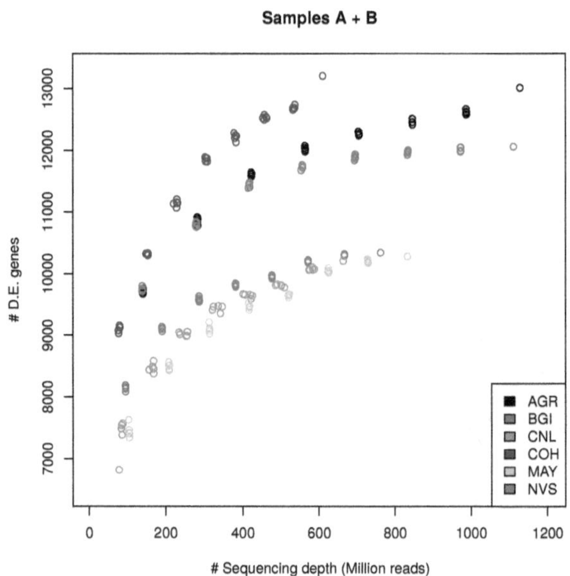

Figure 3.11: The effect in the number of differentially expressed genes in samples A and B in function of the number of lanes being used.

the more differentially expressed genes were detected. Three main groups could be distinguished from the figure. The COH laboratory, which is the one with the largest sequencing depth per replicate, formed the first group, reaching the higher number of differentially expressed genes. However, they sequenced the samples in just one plate. The second group is composed by the AGR and NVS laboratories, which have nearly identical sequencing depth per replicates and number of replicates. Lastly, we find the BGI, CNL and MAY laboratories, which are the ones with the lowest sequencing depths. One thing we found surprising from the results was the lack of a saturation point where the number of DE genes would remain stable despite an increment of the sequencing depth.

3.4.3.4   Transcripts detection

The reproducibility of transcript detection by the RNA-Seq technology was assessed by obtaining the number of transcripts detected with increasing numbers of replicates. The analysis was broken down by expression level intervals to analyse the relationship between consistent detection and expression level as a function of the number of replicates. At each number of replicates and for any given site, all possible combinations of replicates were computed and results were averaged. For example, to compute the number of detected transcripts with 2 replicates in the AGR site (total number of replicates is 4) at the expression range 1-5 fpkm, all combinations of 2 elements out of 4 were generated (6 different combinations). For each combination, the number of transcripts detected simultaneously by the two replicates with expression level within the range 1-5 was computed and values were averaged across all 6 combinations. The analysis was performed for samples A and B, considering both Cufflinks-computed fpkm values and read counts as transcript expression measures.

The average transcript detection values at each cardinality of the replication set were very precise (coefficient of variance typically below 0.01%) and detection patterns were highly consistent across sites provided that uniformity in sequencing depth of replicates was maintained. At low expression values, however, important differences in the number of detected transcripts as a function of the number of replicates were observed (Figure 3.12). For example, at the 0.2-0.5 fpkm range, the number of detected transcripts was reduced on average by a 47% when presence in at least two replicate was required, and 32% and 24% when increasing to three and four replicates. At higher transcript expression values, the robustness of detection was much more stable and in the range 5-10 fpkm, the number of detected transcripts decreased on average by a 17%, 9% and 6% when upgrading to two, three and four replicates, respectively. For all transcript detection ranges, a significant reduction in the number of detected transcripts was observed when the second replicate was introduced. Similar trends could be concluded when considering counts as the measure of transcript expression and trends were also similar for samples A and B across different sites.

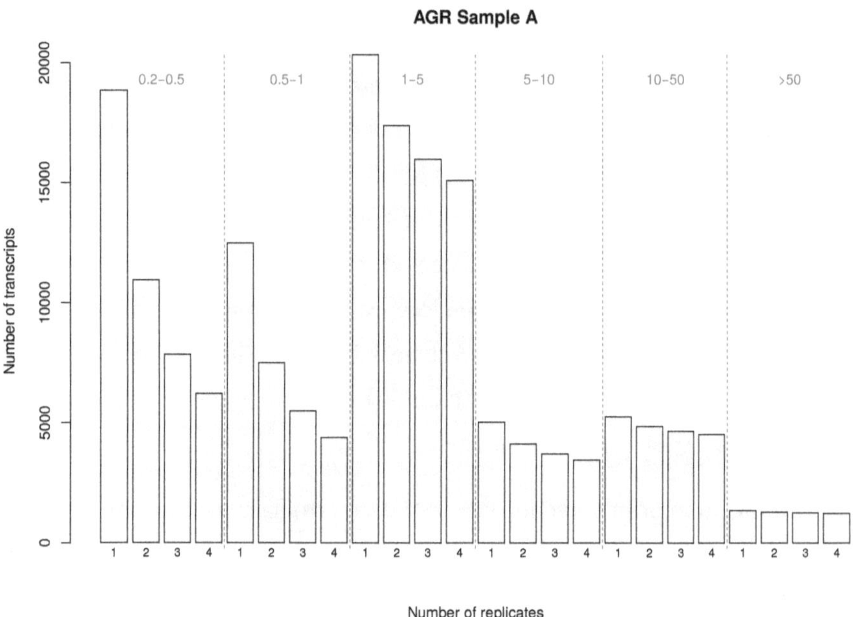

Figure 3.12: The number of transcripts detected by an increasing number of replicates at different transcript expression intervals. Each bar represents the number of transcripts detected simultaneously by at least the indicated number of replicates, averaged through all possible replication sets of that replicates number. Transcripts were identified using Cufflinks and expression measured in FPKM. Data for the AGR site.

These results indicate that transcript detection at low expression levels is strongly noisy and that replication is needed to obtain consistently detected transcripts. At high expression, transcript detection becomes more stable but still, replication helps to control accuracy.

3.4.3.5 *Junctions detection*

The identification and quantification of transcripts from eukaryote genomes based on short read sequencing technologies are coupled to the use of algorithms for transcript inference and expression level estimates. Therefore, the correct prediction of transcript expression is subjected to the accuracy of the algorithm of choice. In order to have a more direct assessment of the ability of RNA-Seq to profile complex transcriptomes consistently, we recorded the detection of reads at exon junctions across replicates and sequencing sites. Junction counts were obtained by extracting from the alignment files those reads that mapped at known exon-exon junction positions. To account for consistency in the detection of alternative splicing events, at each donor site the number of reads mapping at different acceptor sites was obtained, and the percentage of the major alternative junction was calculated as the highest fraction of reads at the acceptor side divided by the total number of reads at the donor side. Only junctions present in the Ensembl annotation were considered. For each sequencing site, we counted the number of junctions detected by at least one to four or five replicates.

Similarly to the transcript detection analysis, a significant reduction of detected junctions was evident as the number of replicates increased. However, only between 10% and 5% of the junctions dropped as the number of replicates raised from 1 to 2, and less than 5% of the remaining junctions were discarded as more replicates were considered (Figure 3.13). It is important to note that the great majority of the detected junctions had no annotated alternative splicing event or these were not found within the mapping data (grey and red colours in stacked bars). However, reads supporting alternative splicing events were in most cases a minority in comparison to the number of reads that supported the most abundant junction (yellow and green stacked bars). This pattern of junction detection was similar for sample A and B, and it was also maintained when looking at junctions detected across different sites, with nearly identical replication yields (i.e. only 1% fewer junctions are detected when inter-site replicates rather than intra-site replicates are considered; Figure 3.14).

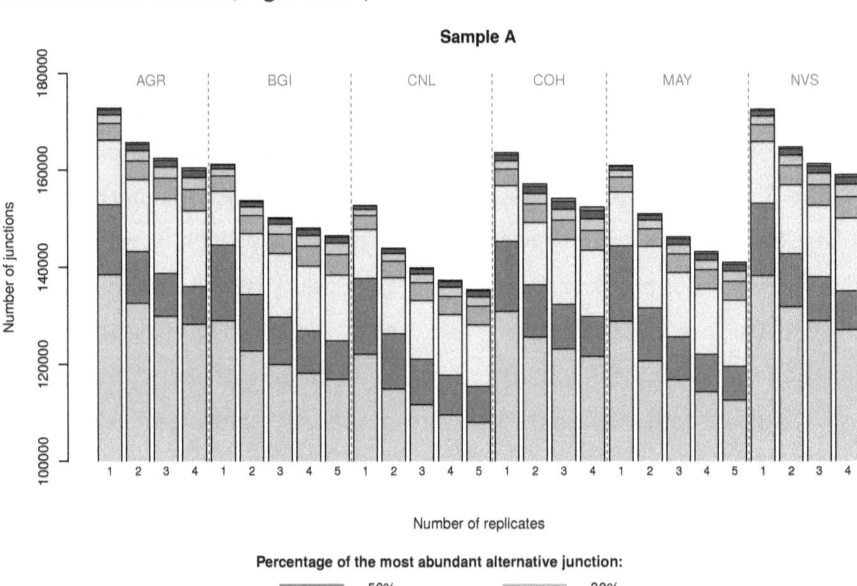

Figure 3.13: The number of junctions detected by an increasing number of replicates at different sequencing sites. Stacked bars indicate the relative frequency of the major junction in case of annotated alternative splicing events at the junction.

Taken together, this analysis suggests that transcript detection fluctuates more than the identification of (alternative) junction sites, especially at the low expression range, and points again to the importance of replication to control the level of false calls.

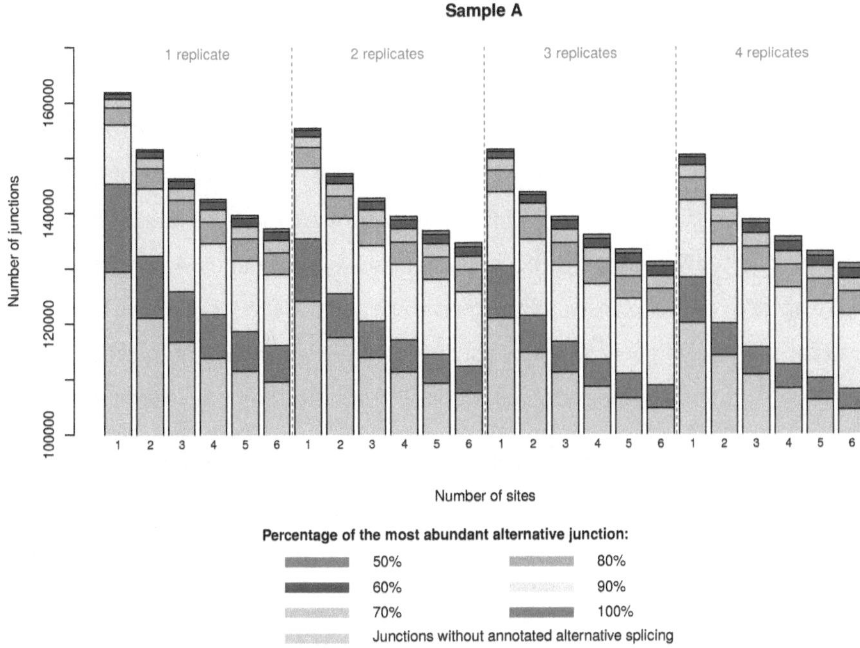

Figure 3.14: The number of junctions detected by Illumina sequencing of sample A across different sequencing sites at different levels of replication. Each bar represents the average number of junctions jointly detected by the indicated number of sites, considering all possible combinations of that site number. For each level of replication, one replication set was randomly selected per site and compared with the replication sets of all remaining sites.

3.5 Discussion

RNA-Seq technology quantifies the number of RNA fragments expressed in a biological sample at a given moment in time. This technology has become the choice of genome-wide transcriptome analysis. However, it is still far from being perfect and researchers are well conscious of the need to perform quality controls over raw and processed data through all the different steps of the processing pipeline to detect and, to some extent, remove any potential technology biases that might arise.

In this chapter, we have presented our efforts to create a Bioconductor R package using the NOISeq algorithm. This package contains a whole set of graphical and diagnostic tools to perform good quality controls over the data. This package was created following the Bioconductor package guidelines. Among those, we were able to reuse the preexisting *ExpressionSet* S4 class to store all the user data and carefully design new S4 classes such as storing the results of the NOISeq algorithm. Additionally, the code was properly structured and user-friendly to run.

Despite performing quality controls is essential for the proper interpretation of downstream analysis, other systemic artefacts might still be present in the data and should be considered before moving forward. One of the most important biases is the sequencing depth effect of the experiment, as we have shown in this chapter. Samples with different sequencing depths cannot be truly comparable and should be corrected prior to analysis. Normalisation methods such as the popular RPKM (Reads Per Kilobase of exon model per Million mapped reads)[36] that normalises the counts by the RNA length applying a division factor of 1 million has been shown to be useful but does not completely remove this bias. In fact, statistical distributions and further analysis might still be affected by the initial coverage difference as we were able to show and as is supported by other work [43, 44]. Notwithstanding, our work was able to show that RNA-Seq technology is extremely robust. The same biological samples were sequenced in different laboratories using the same equipment and the detected bias was always explained by the coverage differences across laboratories. Though this bias can be somehow mitigated, as we have shown during the analyses, it is advisable to avoid this factor from happening to assure all samples have a similar sequencing depth from the first steps.

In the last part of our work, we highlight the importance of working with sample replicates. In our differential expression (DE) analyses, we show how the sequencing depth of a sample vastly affects the detection of differentially expressed genes. Generally, the higher the sequencing depth the more differentially expressed genes will be detected. We also observe how the more replicates we add to the DE analysis, the more DE genes are detected. This is an expected result as the total sequencing depth will increase as we add more replicates to the analysis. We also study the robustness of transcript and junction detection as the number of replicates increases. In particular, for the transcript study, we check the replicability at different RPKM range values. As it might be expected, this analysis can be noisy in lowly covered transcripts (< 1RPKM), so the usage of replicates becomes relevant to obtain consistent results. This detection becomes much more stable in higher expression levels (> 5RPMK) where replicates would not be strictly necessary though they could still be beneficial for better accuracy. These results are supported in [42], where authors show that the higher the sequencing depth, the bigger the diversity and number of detected off-target transcripts. For the junction robustness we took into account for each donor site, which was the acceptor sharing the most reads with this donor as a fraction of the number of reads divided by the total number of reads falling in the donor site. In this case, we found that most of the junctions had no annotated splicing event or these were not found in the mapping data. Besides, the number of junctions detected decreased as replicates were added into the analysis, suggesting we should always have replicates to perform any junction detection analysis to avoid noise and get more accurate results.

Chapter 4

Data integration in NGS

This chapter has been published as:

Furió-Tarí, Pedro, Ana Conesa, and Sonia Tarazona.

RGmatch: Matching Genomic Regions to Proximal Genes in Omics Data Integration.

BMC Bioinformatics 17 (S15): 427. **2016**

4.1   Introduction

The flourishing of sequencing functional genomics assays has popularised the analysis of different chromatin features to elucidate their role on gene expression. These assays measure, for example, the binding of transcription factors or histone modifications at chromosomal locations (chromatin immune precipitation sequencing; ChIP-seq), DNA methylation events (different types of Methyl-seq), or chromatin accessibility (DNase I hypersensitive sites sequencing or Assay for Transposase-Accessible Chromatin with high-throughput sequencing; DNase-seq or ATAC-seq). In all cases, the analysis of this data returns potentially functional regions, defined by genomic coordinates, which must then be related to proximal genes in order to gain any biological meaning. The type of information that can be obtained on the regions regulating nearby genes depends on the type of experiment performed. For example, the transcription factor binding sites predicted using ChIP-seq experiments may be expected to be located in the transcription start site (TSS) and promoter regions of the gene being regulated or in distal enhancers depending whether they are cell-type specific or not, and users might want to have control of what association is relevant in their experiment. In the case of open chromatin sites obtained from DNase-seq experiments, the functional interpretation may differ depending on whether they are in a promoter, intronic, or downstream gene regions. Therefore, it is not only important to associate genomic regions to the closest gene, but also to identify the specific area of the gene where the region is located (the promoter, first exon, an intron, downstream, etc.) [45, 46, 47, 48, 49]. The solution to this problem is not straightforward because it depends on the isoform of the gene being considered. In addition, regions may span multiple areas of the same gene (i.e. the TSS and first exon) or fall at overlapping genes. Moreover, regions at intergenic locations can be associated with upstream or downstream areas of different genes, and therefore a set of rules has to be established to decide which association should be kept.

Because current sequencing technologies predict thousands or even millions of genomic regions that must be mapped to other genomic locations such as genes or transcripts in order to perform integration studies, a computational algorithm is required to match these genomic regions to proximal features (e.g. genes). Moreover, it must take the considerations listed above into account, provide users with flexibility to set the association criteria and be easily integrated with broader analysis pipelines.

Although there is an increasing need for such algorithms, as far as we know, there are very few publicly-available tools which can perform this task. One such tool is part of the HOMER suite [50], which matches each genomic region to the closest transcript and returns the area of the transcript overlapped by the midpoint of the region. This tool can be used with custom annotations, but other information like the overlapping of CpG islands, repeat elements, etc., is only returned for supported species. GREAT [51] is a web tool for predicting *cis*-regulatory regions which takes into account not only nearby genes, but also distal binding events. However, the main drawback of GREAT is its lack of support for species other than human, mouse, and zebrafish. CisGenome [52] is one of the first tools that appeared to deal with ChIP-seq data. Among other utilities, it associates regions to proximal genes but does not provide the location of the region within the gene. This tool can either be used via a graphical interface in Windows operating systems or by command line in OSX and Linux. Seq2pathway [53] and ChIPseeker [54] are two different R packages that also contain functions for associating genomic regions with genes and annotate the location of the region within the gene. Seq2pathway follows a similar approach to GREAT but its main limitation is, again, that it only supports two species (human and mouse). In contrast, ChIPseeker is a more complete tool that supports any species, and which associates regions with the closest gene in a similar way to HOMER.

In this thesis's section we review the main characteristics and drawbacks of some of these tools and present a novel algorithm, RGmatch, to associate genomic regions with proximal features whilst maintaining the flexibility for researchers to set specific match criteria. RGmatch is implemented in Python so it can either be used as a standalone application or incorporated into any omics analysis pipeline. One advantage of RGmatch is its ability to return associations at the gene, transcript, or exon level. The user can deal with the problem of genomic regions overlapping more than one area of a gene (e.g. both the TSS and first exon), by instructing the algorithm to report all the overlapped gene areas (by choosing the exon aggregation level) or by reporting only one association per transcript or per gene, based on a pre-established set of rules. Importantly, these rules, as well as the width of the TSS, promoter, transcription termination site (TTS), or upstream areas, can be modified to meet the researcher's needs.

This work has been developed under the perspective of the STATegra project, an FP7 funded project granted to our group aiming to develop new statistical methods and tools for the integrative analysis of diverse NGS omics data.

4.2   Methods

RGmatch is a rule-based Python software designed to associate genomic regions to genes, transcripts, or exons that also reports the area of the gene where the region overlaps. It requires two essential input files: the genome annotation in GTF format and the chromatin locations of the genomic regions in BED format RGmatch associates each genomic

region with the closest gene (or genes in case of ties resulting from the set of rules used). The distance is computed as the number of bases from the region mid-point to the transcript TSS or TTS. To annotate the area of the transcript where the region falls, we defined eight default disjoint areas (Figure 4.1): TSS, TTS, 1st EXON, PROMOTER, INTRON, GENE BODY, UPSTREAM, and DOWNSTREAM. These areas are defined as follows:

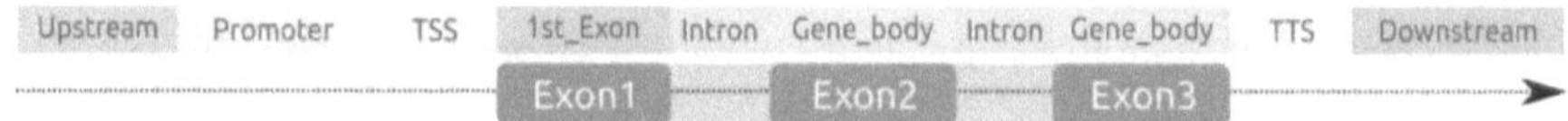

Figure 4.1: Definition of the areas of a gene used by the RGmatch algorithm.

- TSS: Intergenic area adjacent to the TSS point of the gene with a length of t (200 bp by default).

- Promoter: Intergenic area upstream of the TSS with a length of p (1300 bp by default).

- Upstream: Intergenic area upstream of the promoter area, hence more than $t+p$ bp from the TSS point of the gene. This length is limited by the maximum distance, q, allowed by the user, to associate a region with a gene (10 kbp by default).

- 1st_Exon: First exon of the gene.

- Intron: The area between two consecutive exons of a gene.

- Gene_body: The total area of any exon other than the first exon of the gene.

- TTS: Intergenic area adjacent to the TTS point of the gene with a length of s (0 bp by default).

- Downstream: The intergenic area downstream of the TTS area, hence more than s bp from the TTS point of the gene. The length of this area is limited by the maximum distance, q, allowed by the user, between the region and the gene (10 kbp by default).

There are two different cases in which a region could be associated with more than one gene: when two or more genes overlap (Figure 4.2a) or when two (or more) genes are so close ("quasi-overlapping" genes) that the region falls in the overlapping areas of the two genes (Figure 4.2b).

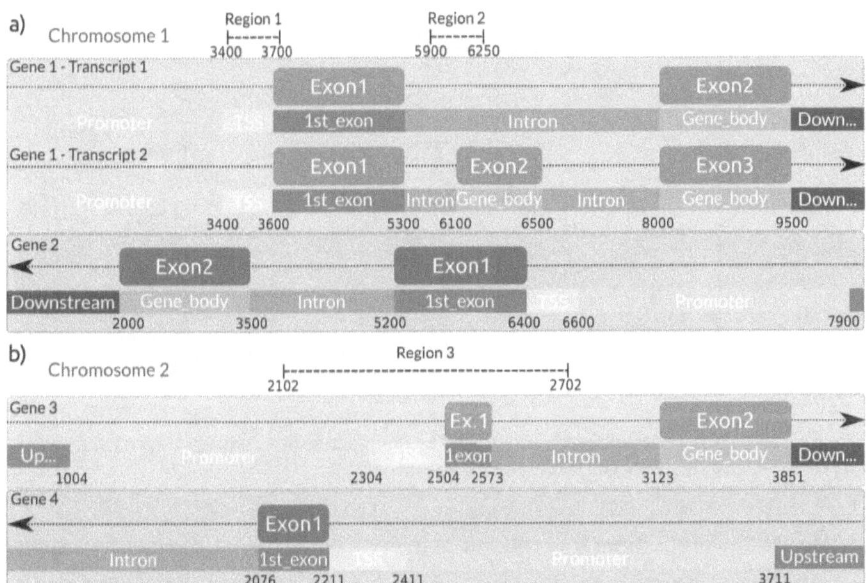

Figure 4.2: Examples of two different situations that would result in a region being associated with more than one gene. **a** Two overlapped genes with different isoforms. **b** Two different genes with common areas overlapping the region (quasi-overlapping genes)

When the region overlaps several areas of a gene but the user needs to choose a single area per gene or transcript to annotate the association, a set of rules has to be defined in order to select the most appropriate one. The rules defined by

RGmatch are based on the percentage of the region overlapping each area of the gene ("*PercRegion*"), the percentage of each gene area that is overlapped by the region ("*PercArea*"), and a rank of priorities for the areas to be used in the case of any ties (by default: TSS, 1st EXON, PROMOTER, TTS, INTRON, GENE BODY, UP-STREAM, DOWNSTREAM). As summarised in Figure 4.3, if there is an area for which *PercRegion* $\geq$ w (50 % by default), this area will be the annotation for that region-transcript association. Otherwise, the algorithm uses the area with *PercArea* $\geq$ v (90 % by default).

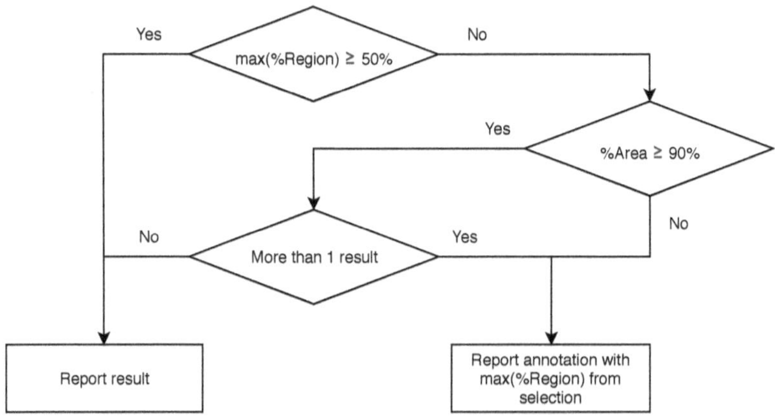

Figure 4.3: Flowchart describing the rules used by RGmatch to decide the gene area to annotate the region-transcript association (default algorithm options)

When several areas meet this condition, the one with highest *PercRegion* is selected. In the case of ties, the selected area is determined according to the list of priorities. The default percentages to apply the rules (v and w) and the default area priorities can be easily modified by the user.

One of the main advantages of RGmatch is its ability to report the associations at different aggregation levels (exon, transcript, or gene). By default, it reports all possible associations to the different areas of the exons. When choosing the report at the 'transcript aggregation level', the algorithm applies the set of previously-defined rules in order to return a single area per region and transcript. The same rules apply when reporting at the 'gene aggregation level', but in this case, if the region is located in different areas for each transcript of a given gene, the rank of priorities will be used to annotate the association to only one of them.

RGmatch generates a tabular text output file with the following columns:

- **Region:** Identifier (ID) of the region being associated. This ID is generated by RGmatch and consists of the chromosome, start and end positions, separated by an underscore (chr_start_end).

- **Midpoint:** Midpoint of the region being associated.

- **Gene:** Gene ID for the gene that has been associated to the region.

- **Transcript:** Transcript ID for the transcript that has been associated to the region. When reporting at the gene aggregation level the algorithm will report all the possible transcripts in the case of internal ties.

- **Exon:** Exon number associated to the region. In the case of transcript ties, when reporting at gene aggregation level, the value reported will be -1.

- **Area:** Area of the gene (or transcript) where the region falls.

- **Distance:** Distance from the TSS or TTS to the midpoint of the region. When the region overlaps a gene, the distance reported is 0.

- **PercRegion:** Percentage of the region that overlaps the area of the gene reported.

- **PercArea:** Percentage of the reported area overlapped by the region.

- If the input BED file has more columns than the three mandatory ones, these columns are attached in the output file after the *PercArea* column.

The associations rendered by RGmatch at the three different aggregation levels for the two examples shown in Figure 4.2, according to the rules described and using the default parameters, are shown in Tables 4.1, 4.2 and 4.3, and to illustrate how the algorithm works some of them are also described below.

Region	Midpoint	Gene	Transcript	Exon	Area	Distance	PercRegion	PercArea
1_3400_3700	3550	Gene2	Tr1_Gene2	2	INTRON	0	66.45	-1
1_3400_3700	3550	Gene2	Tr1_Gene2	2	GENE_BODY	0	33.55	6.73
1_3400_3700	3550	Gene1	Tr1_Gene1	1	TSS	0	66.45	100.0
1_3400_3700	3550	Gene1	Tr1_Gene1	1	1st_EXON	0	33.55	5.94
1_3400_3700	3550	Gene1	Tr2_Gene1	1	TSS	0	66.45	100.0
1_3400_3700	3550	Gene1	Tr2_Gene1	1	1st_EXON	0	33.55	5.94
1_5900_6250	6075	Gene2	Tr1_Gene2	1	1st_EXON	0	100	29.23
1_5900_6250	6075	Gene1	Tr2_Gene1	2	INTRON	0	56.98	-1
1_5900_6250	6075	Gene1	Tr2_Gene1	2	GENE_BODY	0	43.02	37.66
2_2102_2702	2402	Gene4	Tr1_Gene4	1	TSS	0	33.28	100.0
2_2102_2702	2402	Gene4	Tr1_Gene4	1	PROMOTER	0	48.42	22.38
2_2102_2702	2402	Gene4	Tr1_Gene4	1	1st_EXON	0	18.30	80.88
2_2102_2702	2402	Gene3	Tr1_Gene3	1	TSS	0	33.28	100.0
2_2102_2702	2402	Gene3	Tr1_Gene3	1	PROMOTER	0	33.61	15.54
2_2102_2702	2402	Gene3	Tr1_Gene3	1	1st_EXON	0	11.65	100
2_2102_2702	2402	Gene3	Tr1_Gene3	1	INTRON	0	21.46	-1

Table 4.1: Table showing the results at the exon level for the example shown in Figure 4.2

Region 1 (1_3400_3700) from Figure 4.2a overlaps Gene 1 and Gene 2. Gene 1 has two different transcripts. If we report at the exon level, RGmatch returns all the areas of the different genes overlapped by the region. In this example, Region 1 overlaps the entire 'TSS' (100 %) and part of the '1st_exon' (5.94 %) of both transcripts of Gene 1, and part of the 'gene_body' and 'intron' areas of Gene 2. RGmatch reports the different overlap percentages, except for introns (for which

Region	Midpoint	Gene	Transcript	Exon	Area	Distance	PercRegion	PercArea
1_3400_3700	3550	Gene1	Tr2_Gene1	1	TSS	0	66.45	100.0
1_3400_3700	3550	Gene2	Tr1_Gene2	1	INTRON	0	66.45	-1
1_3400_3700	3550	Gene1	Tr1_Gene1	1	TSS	0	66.45	100.0
1_5900_6250	6075	Gene1	Tr2_Gene1	1	INTRON	0	56.98	-1
1_5900_6250	6075	Gene2	Tr1_Gene2	1	1st_EXON	0	100	29.23
2_2102_2702	2402	Gene4	Tr1_Gene4	1	TSS	0	33.28	100.0
2_2102_2702	2402	Gene3	Tr1_Gene3	1	TSS	0	33.28	100.0

Table 4.2: Table showing the results at the transcript level for the example shown in Figure 4.2

Region	Midpoint	Gene	Transcript	Exon	Area	Distance	PercRegion	PercArea
1_3400_3700	3550	Gene1	Tr2_Gene1_Tr1_Gene1	-1	TSS	-1	-1	-1
1_3400_3700	3550	Gene2	Tr1_Gene2	1	INTRON	0	66.45	-1
1_5900_6250	6075	Gene1	Tr2_Gene1	1	INTRON	0	56.98	1
1_5900_6250	6075	Gene2	Tr1_Gene2	1	1st_EXON	0	100	29.23
2_2102_2702	2402	Gene3	Tr1_Gene3	1	TSS	0	33.28	100.0
2_2102_2702	2402	Gene4	Tr1_Gene4	1	TSS	0	33.28	100.0

Table 4.3: Table showing the results at the gene level for the example shown in Figure 4.2

it returns a -1 result). Of the total length of Region 1, 66 % overlaps the 'TSS' of Gene 1 (for both transcripts) and the 'intron' of Gene 2. According to the previously described rules, given that this percentage is higher than the 50 % set as threshold, these areas will be returned when reporting at the transcript level (Table 4.2). In the gene-level report, both Gene1 and Gene2 are associated with Region 1 (overlapping genes). For Gene1, the association is annotated to 'TSS' since both transcripts had the same annotation.

Region 3 from Figure 4.2b overlaps Gene 3 and Gene 4, and has a percentage of overlap of 33.28, 33.61, 11.65, and 21.46 % with the 'TSS', 'promoter', '1st_exon', and 'intron' regions of Gene 3, respectively. When reporting at the transcript or gene aggregation levels, since these overlap percentages do not exceed 50 % in any case, we have to look at the percentage of each gene area overlapped by the region. Two different areas ('TSS' and '1st_exon') are completely overlapped with a percentage higher than 90 %, and so they are tied. In this case, the algorithm returns the area with the highest percentage of the region overlapping it, which corresponds to the TSS (33.28 %). The same procedure also has to be applied to Gene 4, this process results in the same TSS annotation. Therefore, Region 3 will have two associated genes reported with the 'TSS' annotation (quasi-overlapping genes).

RGmatch provides many configuration options and the user can modify the priorities and rules followed to associate a region with a gene area. The following arguments can be optionally set by the user:

- **Report**: Argument to select the aggregation level for the report. By default, it is set to 'exon' and all possible associations to all the different areas of a gene or genes where the region overlaps will be reported. When it is set to 'transcript' or 'gene' the rules explained above are applied.

- **Distance**: By default, a region will be associated to a gene if it is closer than 10 kbp.

- **TSS**: Area starting at the transcription start site of a gene and finishing t bp upstream from that point. By default, $t = 200$.

- **TTS**: Intergenic area starting at the transcription termination site of a gene with a length of s bp. By default, $s = 0$, so this area is not considered unless this parameter is modified by the user.

- **Promoter**: Area starting one nucleotide after the predefined TSS area and extending up to p bp upstream from that point. By default, $p = 1300$.

- **PercArea**: Threshold for the percentage of the gene area overlapped by the region, used in the selection rules (see flowchart in Figure 4.3). By default, this is set at 90 %.

- **PercRegion**: Threshold for the percentage of the region overlapping the gene area, used in the selection rules (see flowchart in Figure 4.3). By default, this is set at 50 %.

- **Rules**: In case of ties after following the rules shown in Figure 4.3, the algorithm will decide the area to annotate the association to according to a rank of priorities. By default, this is: TSS, 1st_EXON, PROMOTER, TTS, INTRON, GENE_BODY, UPSTREAM, and DOWNSTREAM. To modify these priorities, a string containing the eight disjoint areas must be introduced.

- **Gene**: Tag indicating which gene identifier from the GTF annotation file is to be reported. By default 'gene_id' is used.

- **Transcript**: Tag indicating which transcript identifier from the GTF annotation file is to be reported. By default 'transcript_id' is used.

- **GTF**: Mandatory input. GTF annotation file. Files compressed with gzip are also accepted.

- **BED**: Mandatory input. BED file with the set of genomic regions to be matched. Files compressed with gzip are also accepted.

- **Output**: Mandatory input. Full path and name of the file where the output will be written.

4.3   Results and discussion

In order to show the functionalities and main advantages of RGmatch, we compared it to the other methods available: HOMER, GREAT, CisGenome, Seq2pathway, and ChIPseeker. Comparisons are difficult because, on the one hand, there is no gold-standard data set of true associations between the genomic regions and the genes and, on the other hand, the goal of the different methods is not always exactly the same. For instance, GREAT and Seq2pathway do not only return the closest gene but also other distal genes by following an approach that is completely different from the other methods. GREAT assigns a 'regulatory domain' for each gene, so if any region lies within the regulatory domain, it is assumed to regulate the gene. There are three options to define this regulatory domain. The default option (the one we compared RGmatch to), called the 'basal plus extension', assigns a 'basal regulatory region' that extends 5 kbp upstream and 1 kbp downstream of the TSS, irrespective of the presence of any neighbouring genes. Based on a similar approach, Seq2pathway takes the functional impact of coding and non-coding genes into account to make associations. In the following sections, we provide both qualitative and quantitative comparisons based on the results obtained with a publicly available set of genomic regions.

4.3.1   *Qualitative comparison to the state-of-the-art methods*

In this section, we highlight the characteristics of RGmatch that make it different from any of the other approaches (see a summary in Table 4.4), and which therefore support the need to make this novel tool available to the research community.

	RGmatch	HOMER	GREAT	CisGenome	Seq2pathway	ChIPseeker
User-friendly	Command line	Command line	Web tool	Command line/GI (only in Windows)	R/Bioc	R/Bioc
Adaptable to pipelines	Yes	Yes[a]	No	Yes[a]	Yes[a]	Yes[a]
Input format	BED (also gzip-compressed BED file)	BED	BED (only 3 columns)	BED -> COD	BED -> GRanges	BED
Association resolution	Gene, transcript, exon	Gene, transcript	Gene	Gene	Gene	Gene, transcript
Area annotation	Yes	Yes	No	No	Yes	Yes
Flexibility	Distance, Areas, Rules, Area priorities	No	Distance	Distance	Search radius	Area priorities, TSS distance
Supported species	All	All	3	12	2	All[b]
Output: Gene IDs?	Any in the GTF	Gene and transcript IDs	Gene names	Gene IDs	Gene IDs and gene names	Gene and transcript IDs
Output: Distance?	Yes	Yes	Yes	No	Yes	Yes
Output: Overlapping genes?	Yes	No	No	No	Yes	No

[a] HOMER and CisGenome can be integrated in analysis pipelines, although the process to obtain the annotations and parse these results is not as straightforward as with RGmatch. Seq2pathway and ChIPseeker can also be integrated with additional scripting.
[b] It supports all species, provided the input format is a TxDb R object. This format can be obtained from a GTF file by using the *makeTxDbFromGFF* function in the GenomicFeatures package.

Table 4.4: Comparison of the functionalities of the different algorithms

4.3.1.1 User-friendly

RGmatch and HOMER are easy-to-use command line algorithms that can be run locally on any computer and in any operating system provided Python or Perl interpreters are installed. GREAT is accessible via their website, which makes it user-friendly on any operating system, but it cannot be used locally. CisGenome can also be used in any operating system via command line and has a graphical interface, but only for Windows. On the contrary, ChIPseeker and Seq2pathway are both R packages that can be easily used if the R interpreter is installed. However, we had problems using Seq2pathway on the Linux platform because the association function did not work.

4.3.1.2 Adaptable to pipelines

All methods except GREAT, which is a web tool, can be easily integrated into any analysis pipeline. HOMER is a suite of tools, and the whole suite has to be installed for the method to work. As for all R packages, ChIPSeeker and Seq2pathway, can also be integrated into any analysis pipeline, although some additional scripting is required. In contrast, RGmatch can be directly used in any pipeline and does not require additional steps or modules to work.

4.3.1.3 Input format

RGmatch, GREAT, HOMER, and ChIPSeeker take a BED file containing the regions to be associated as input. CisGenome and Seq2pathway require the BED file to be converted into their own formats. GREAT accepts a 3-column BED file. The other methods accept BED files containing information other than genome coordinates, but only RGmatch and ChIPSeeker return the additional columns in the output file.

4.3.1.4 Association resolution

A unique feature of RGmatch is its ability to report associations at the exon, transcript, or gene level. GREAT, CisGenome, and Seq2pathway only report associations at the gene level, whereas HOMER and ChIPSeeker can report associations at the gene or transcript level.

4.3.1.5   Location of the region

RGmatch, HOMER, Seq2pathway, and ChIPSeeker report the area of the gene where the region overlaps for each association. Neither GREAT nor CisGenome return this information.

4.3.1.6   Flexibility

RGmatch, CisGenome, Seq2pathway, and GREAT let users modify the basic parameters (related to the maximum distance) used to associate a region to a gene. HOMER, on the contrary, always associates the region to a gene no matter how far it is. RGmatch and ChIPSeeker also allow the user to modify the length of some gene areas, as well as the priorities for annotating the association with the gene area. In addition, RGmatch offers a flexible definition of the association rules, while this is not possible in HOMER or Seq2pathway.

4.3.1.7   Supported species

RGmatch, HOMER, and ChIPseeker work with any organism as long as the user provides the GTF annotation file. However, ChIPseeker requires the annotations to be converted to TxDb[1] R objects beforehand. GREAT, Seq2pathway, and Cis-Genome only work with the species list they provide; at the moment, GREAT and Seq2pathway both support 4 species, whereas CisGenome supports 12.

---

[1] The TxDb class is an R container for storing transcript annotations.

4.3.1.8 Output

All of the algorithms compared return a tabulated file containing the region-gene associations and some additional information. Only RGmatch and ChIPSeeker preserve the original columns in the BED file when more than the three mandatory columns containing the genomic positions are provided (e.g. coverage, quality, *p*-values, etc. may also be included in the region BED file). RGmatch also allows the user to choose the gene identifier to be reported among all the identifiers in the GTF file. In HOMER and ChIPseeker, the user can choose between gene and transcript IDs, CisGenome reports the gene ID, and GREAT returns gene names. All the methods except CisGenome report the distance between the gene and the region. RGmatch, HOMER, ChIPseeker, and Seq2pathway return the area of the gene overlapped by the region. The gene area definitions are similar for HOMER, ChIPseeker, and RGmatch, or at least they can be made almost equivalent by tuning the RGmatch parameters. However, the column containing the gene area in the HOMER and ChIPseeker outputs also contains additional information so this column cannot be directly used in further analyses where a categorical classification of the gene areas is needed unless it is properly parsed first. Another unique feature of RGmatch and Seq2pathway is that if a region can be associated with two or more overlapping genes, all of them are reported as different rows in the output file, while the other methods only provide one associated gene in these cases.

4.3.1.9 Quantitative comparison

To quantitatively assess the functionality of our approach, we compared RGmatch to HOMER and CisGenome using a public set of genomic regions. We discarded GREAT and Seq2pathway from the comparison because they follow a completely different approach to associate chromatin regions, meaning that the results are not directly comparable. We also decided not to include ChIPseeker because it is very similar to HOMER. The public set of genomic regions used in the comparison contained 2638 regions from a human ChIP-Seq experiment, and was downloaded from the Sequence Read Archive (SRA) with accession number GSE55727. The annotation (GTF file) was downloaded from Ensembl GRCh37.75.

In order to make the outputs comparable between the methods, the RGmatch report was performed at the gene aggregation level, the maximum distance for reporting associations was set to 1000 kbp to allow at least one association per region, the promoter length was set to 0, and the TSS area was set to 1kbp. The rest of the parameters were left at their default values. We used the default parameters for HOMER. To run CisGenome, first the GTF was converted to refFlat format using the *gtfToGenePred* tool from the University of California Santa Cruz Genomics Institute, and then the BED file was converted to COD format using the *file_bed2cod* tool provided by CisGenome. CisGenome was then run setting the distance limits to 1000 kbp and leaving the rest of the parameters at their default values. Regions corresponding to chromosomes X and Y were removed from the BED file used for all of the algorithms because CisGenome does not take them into account, which left a total of 2592 regions.

Each of the final 2592 regions was associated with a single gene by HOMER and CisGenome. RGmatch returned 3406 associations due to overlapping and quasi-overlapping genes. The percentage of common associations reported by the three methods was high (Figure 4.4). Over 85% of the associations called by RGmatch were also reported by HOMER and/or CisGenome. However, RGmatch reported 739 associations that were not called by the other two methods. Most of them (731) were due to the fact that RGmatch can associate regions to two different genes, so one of the two genes is reported by the other two methods, but the second gene is only reported by RGmatch. The reason for the remaining 8 associations, that were exclusively detected by RGmatch, was because RGmatch associated the region to the closest gene (which was downstream), while HOMER associated it to a more distal gene in an upstream area. There is no clear reason why CisGenome returned a different association for these cases. The associations that were common to RGmatch and only one of the other two methods were generally also due to RGmatch associating the region to two overlapping (or quasi-overlapping) genes whereas HOMER reported one of the two associations and CisGenome reported the other.

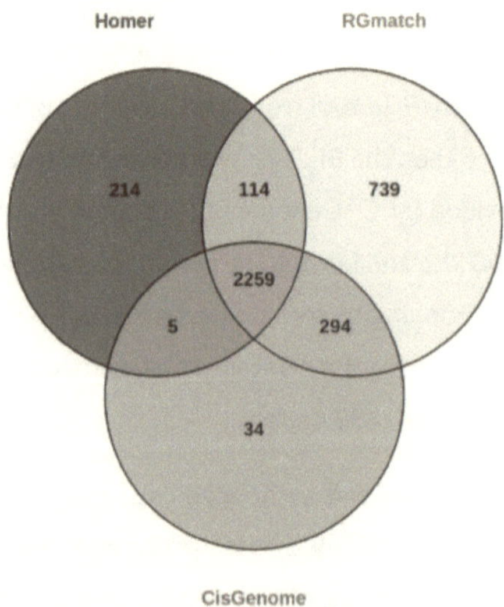

Figure 4.4: Venn diagram showing the number of region-gene associations obtained with the HOMER, RGmatch, and CisGenome methods

We also observed that, in some cases where the methods returned different results, the associated region was far away from the genes. RGmatch associated the region to the closest gene, even if the region was downstream from the gene. In these cases, CisGenome tends to associate the region to a gene with an upstream annotation (even if it is not the closest gene), while HOMER either does the same or chooses a downstream annotation but to the second closest gene.

RGmatch and HOMER also report the area of the gene where the region overlaps. However, the definition of the gene areas reported by these two methods is not exactly the same. HOMER defines their 'promoter-TSS' as the region comprising -1 kbp to +100 bp from the start of the gene and the 'TTS' as the region comprising from -100 bp to +1 kbp from the end of the gene. In order to cover the same areas, we defined our 'TSS' area as -1 kbp to -1 bp and removed the 'promoter' area. This way, HOMER's TSS area was equivalent to ours plus the first 100 bps from our '1st_exon' area, and our 'Downstream' area was equivalent to Homer's TTS and Intergenic area, etc. (see all the equivalences in Table 4.5).

RGmatch	HOMER
INTRON	Intron
UPSTREAM	Intergenic
DOWNSTREAM	TTS; Intergenic
GENE_BODY	exon; 3' UTR; 5' UTR
TSS	promoter-TSS
1st_EXON	exon; promoter-TSS; 5' UTR; 3' UTR

Table 4.5: Equivalences between the gene areas defined by RGmatch and HOMER

Table 4.6 shows the number of associations reported by HOMER and RGmatch with equivalent annotations for the region location (in green), accounting for the vast majority (more than 95% of the reported associations). Associations, where the gene area did not agree, are indicated in red. Discrepancies are due to regions overlapping several areas of the gene. In such cases, the true location of the region in the gene is unclear. While HOMER chooses the area overlapping the midpoint of the region, the RGmatch annotation is based on the overlap percentage and on the priorities chosen by the user, allowing them to fine-tune the association results depending on their analysis goals.

		RGmatch						
		UPSTREAM	INTRON	DOWNSTREAM	TSS	TTS	1st_Exon	GENE_BODY
HOMER	intron		1246					1
	Intergenic	440		341				
	exon		14				24	20
	promoter-TSS		1		171	1	23	
	TTS					104	3	6
	5' UTR		1				4	
	3' UTR							12

Associations with equal or equivalent annotations in both methods are shown in green, and associations with different annotations are shown in red

Table 4.6: Annotations for the region location within the gene returned by RGmatch (columns) and HOMER (rows)

In summary, the association results from RGmatch are comparable to the results provided by other methods. Nevertheless, RGmatch is more flexible than other approaches because it allows to define the rules to compute the associations and annotate them with the region location within the gene. Moreover, it returns all the possible associations when the region overlaps more than one gene (overlapping or quasioverlapping genes), and the output is easier for the user to understand and re-use.

To check the efficiency of the algorithms, we compared the computation time and memory used when running the algorithms on the full human ChIP-seq example (2638 regions, including the X and Y chromosomes) with the human reference genome annotation GTF file. RGmatch took 32 seconds to obtain the results and required 1 GB of RAM memory. In contrast, HOMER took 1 minute and 30 seconds and required up to 3 GB of RAM. CisGenome was almost instantaneous, since it requires a prior transformation of the input files. These calculations were performed on an Intel(R) Xeon(R) CPU E3-1225 V2 @ 3.20GHz machine.

RGmatch was designed to check only the proximal annotations for each region. This implies that it is highly scalable despite having a large number of regions. In our tests, RGmatch obtained results in 15 s using a file with 25,000 regions, 50 s with 200,000 regions and 122 s with 600,000 regions in a 2.4 GHz Intel Core i5. The slowest step is the internal ordering of the regions and annotations, but the association step is straightforward.

4.4 Conclusions

As sequencing technologies evolve and studies that integrate gene expression with chromatin features become more common, the need to associate genomic regions to genes in order to understand regulatory mechanisms has increased. Although there are a number of publicly available tools to perform this task, most of them have limitations in terms of flexibility or usability.

In this work, we present RGmatch, a user-friendly tool for matching genomic regions and genes, transcripts or exons, which reports the area of the gene where the region overlaps. RGmatch supports all species as long as the user provides the GTF file with the reference genome annotation. The tool is a freely accessible Python script, which promotes integration into broader analysis pipelines. RGmatch is a valuable resource for facilitating analysis in multi-omics experiments involving gene expression and different types of chromatin features.

The main advantages of RGmatch, when compared to the state-of-the-art methods, are the flexibility for the user to define its association rules, gene areas, gene identifiers to be reported, and priorities for the gene area annotation when the region overlaps different areas of the gene, as well as its ability to report associations at different aggregation levels. In addition, when a genomic region overlaps several genes, all the associations are returned. Therefore, RGmatch provides a biologically meaningful set of rules and parameters that can be tuned by users to adapt the associations to their preferences or needs.

Chapter 5

Functional characterisation of long non-coding RNAs

Part of this chapter has been published as:

<u>Furió-Tarí, Pedro</u>, Sonia Tarazona, Toni Gabaldón, Anton J. Enright, and Ana Conesa.

spongeScan: A Web for Detecting MicroRNA Binding Elements in LncRNA Sequences.

Nucleic Acids Research (Oxford University Press) 44 (W1): W176–80. **2016**

5.1   Introduction

Next Generation Sequencing technologies and in particular RNA-Seq brought new information on genome organisation. One of the most exciting discoveries of NGS is that a large proportion of the genome is transcribed into RNAs with an apparent lack of coding potential [13, 14, 15]. Long non-coding RNAs (lncRNAs) are defined as non-coding RNA transcripts longer than 200 nucleotides [17, 18, 19, 20]. They are particularly known for being expressed in a few specific tissues only acting as important gene regulators through different mechanisms [21]. They have been shown to regulate transcription modulating the chromatin by binding histone-modifying complexes [55], binding the RNA Polymerase II directly to inhibit transcription [23] by forming lncRNA-DNA triplex structures that inhibit the formation of the preinitiation complex [24] or even by folding into structures that mimic other DNA-binding sites or inhibit or enhance the activity of other specific transcription factors [56, 57], among others.

At the time this work was performed, few publications had studied the impact of some lncRNAs in different kind of cancer types such as HOTAIR in breast [58], MALAT1 in lung [59] or HULC in liver [60]. However, genome-wide analyses integrating data from different tissues and conditions with the goal of predicting lncRNA functions were missing. The guilty by association approach is widely used to infer functions of genes which remain unknown. This relies on the idea that any non-described genes associated or interacting with any described genes are very likely to share functions or pathways. In this chapter, we will use this approach to look for co-expression patterns between lncRNAs and protein-coding genes. To do so, we will use the Gene Ontology (GO) knowledgebase as the main source of information of the protein-coding gene functions. GO terms explain how individual genes contribute to the biology of an organism at the molecular, cellular and organism levels. Therefore, GO annotations should be a good resource to functionally annotate lncRNAs.

Other ways of inferring functions of lncRNAs are more related to the sequence structure and the molecular interaction prediction. LncRNAs are also known to sequester miRNAs inhibiting their functions. In this chapter, we will also present the application of this strategy in the way of a web application to help find non-coding transcripts harbouring miRNA response elements (MREs) where miRNAs bind.

5.2   Objectives

The work described in this chapter aims to create a methodology for the functional annotation of long non-coding RNAs as well as a web resource to predict lncRNAs harbouring MREs.

For the first development, High-Performance Computing approaches developed for NGS analysis in our department were used to conduct a large-scale computational analysis of RNA-Seq datasets present in public repositories. The strategy was to analyse co-expression patterns of lncRNAs with annotated protein-coding genes among a wide number of experimental conditions to find strong correlation patterns between the coding and non-coding genes and use these, through appropriate algorithms, to identify functional categories which can be assigned to the so far uncharacterised lncRNAs (guilty-by-association).

For the second part, we sought to develop a novel, sequence-based, algorithm designed for the detection of MREs in non-coding transcripts that have the potential to act as competing endogenous RNAs (ceRNAs) of miRNAs. This algorithm would be potentially applicable to any organism where sequence data is available. We will also describe a new web resource, spongeScan, which provides a user-friendly interface for applying this sponge search algorithm to any set of sequences provided by the user. spongeScan also includes options to analyse gene expression data of both candidate ceRNAs and miRNAs. It is important to mention that spongeScan does not give a definitive prediction value, but rather ranks putative ceRNA–miRNAs pairs on the basis of several parameters that are indicative of sponge function [27]. Our algorithm particularly identifies lncRNAs that have multiple and spread MREs.

5.3   Functional characterisation of long non-coding RNAs

5.3.1   *Methods*

Data retrieval

In order to develop the new methodology for lncRNA functional annotation, data were downloaded from public repositories. These data had to meet the following criteria:

1. be annotated as *Homo sapiens* species.

2. sequencing depth between 50 and 80 million reads. Samples with lower sequencing depths were also considered as long as there were replicates that could be joined to achieve a minimum sequencing depth.

3. data has to be sequenced on Illumina platforms.

4. cover as many tissues and cell lines as possible trying to achieve a balance among them.

5. preference for paired-end data. However, single-end data with high quality was also acceptable.

Data were retrieved from the ENCODE project as well as from the Sequence Read Archive (SRA). Samples obtained from ENCODE were taken from the "RNA-Seq from ENCODE/Caltech" and "Long RNA-Seq from ENCODE/Cold Spring Harbor Lab" studies.

A total of 206 samples were downloaded (54 samples from the SRA, 34 samples from ENCODE/Caltech and 118 samples from ENCODE/Cold Spring Harbor).

Preprocessing

Quality control of the *fastq* files of the samples was performed using the FastQC[6] software. Four different groups of samples were found based on their qualities:

1. samples with an overall good quality were kept for following analyses;

2. samples with extremely bad qualities were discarded from our final dataset;

3. samples with low quality in the last nucleotides were trimmed as long as the resulting length would be higher than 30bps, otherwise discarded;

4. samples with quality drops across the whole length of the reads were treated differently.

A quality threshold was applied using a minimum *Phred Score* of 20, which stands for a base accuracy of 99%. This was performed using the filtering tool FastX toolkit[61], which checks the reads backwards starting trimming from the last nucleotide of each read. Whenever it finds a nucleotide with a *Phred Score* over the indicated threshold, it stops trimming. However, this approach leads to additional problems when applied to paired-end data. This is because some reads might be completely discarded while the pair might still be valid leaving this last one as an "orphan" read. In order to rescue these "orphan" reads and have the biggest coverage possible, a custom Python script was developed to remove them from the pair-end fastq file and to pull them into a different single-end fastq file. From this point on, paired-end data as well as single-end orphan reads, were treated in a different way. Sequencing depth was checked again after the read correction and samples with less than 50 million reads were filtered out, unless there was a biological replicate with also a low number of reads. In those cases, samples were merged to reach the targeted sequencing depth requirements.

Reads were mapped using TopHat[41] v2.0.8 against the University of California Santa Cruz (UCSC) hg19 assembly reference genome. Single-end data, as well as paired-end data with no filtering issues were mapped as usual. Samples containing paired-end reads as well as orphan reads, were mapped using the following strategy: TopHat builds a junctions file every time the mapping process is performed, containing all the junctions that have been found during the mapping step. Because the number of orphan reads was much lower than the number of paired-end reads, and the single-end approach is noisier, paired-end reads were mapped as usual first, and the junctions file built during the previous mapping step was used to help the mapping process of the orphan reads. In the end, two different BAM files were obtained for every filtered paired-end sample. Samples with an extremely low proportion of mapped reads were filtered out at this point.

Two different approaches were evaluated for quantifying gene expression from BAM files: HTSeq and Qualimap. HTSeq 0.5.3p3[62] only takes into account reads mapping to only one location in the genome. Reads mapping to different features (multihits) were not considered. However, there were other tools that could take multihits into account. Qualimap[9], for example, had two different approaches implemented for these cases: (i) count each read as if it was uniquely mapped; or (ii) count reads mapping to different locations in a proportional way. However, Qualimap was limited at the moment of this analysis because it considered paired-end reads as if they were single-end, so the number of counts would be duplicated for some reads, and therefore, not really trustworthy. In an attempt to get the best of both approaches, a Python script was developed to implement the proportional approach using HTSeq. This script performed the following steps:

1. split each BAM file into several BAM files, each one containing only reads mapping to 1 feature, 2 features, etc.;

2. modify the FLAG[1] for each read to make HTSeq to recode the read as single hit;

3. run in parallel as many HTSeq processes as BAM files were generated;

4. counts obtained after running HTSeq with the BAM file containing reads mapping to 2 different features were divided by 2, the ones obtained after running it with the BAM file with reads mapping to 3 different features were divided by 3, etc.;

5. generate one single count file adding up the counts of the different files.

The counting step was performed for all the samples using that script. This was performed twice for the filtered paired-end samples, one with the BAM file obtained after mapping the paired-end reads and other with the BAM obtained after mapping the orphan reads. The counts obtained with each of the files were finally added up. In the end, a total of 161 samples were used for further analysis.

---

[1] Combination of bitwise flags that describe different properties of the mapped read.

Due to the heterogeneity of the data, counts were normalised by the effective sequencing depth. Additional metadata information was added to the count matrix such as the laboratory or tissue where each sample came or was taken from. Additionally, genes were categorised as protein-coding or long non-coding genes. Data was checked for any possible bias and corrected using ASCA-genes, an R package developed in our group that is an adaptation of the ASCA method (ANOVA Simultaneous Component Analysis) to the analysis of multifactorial experiments in transcriptomics

Functional annotation

A guilty-by-association approach was considered to functionally annotate lncRNAs. To do so, lncRNAs were grouped into two different groups: tissue and non-tissue-specific lncRNAs. To group lncRNAs, the following *tau* formula [5.1][63] was used:

$$\tau = \frac{\sum_{i=1}^{N}(1 - x_i)}{N - 1} \tag{5.1}$$

In this formula, the N was considered as the number of tissues, x_i the expression level of the lncRNA in tissue i normalised by the maximal expression level in the N tissues. The described formula returns a value between 0 and 1 for each gene. Values closer to 1 would be returned for genes expressed in just a few samples (tissue-specific) and closer to 0 when expressed in almost all the samples (non-specific).

However, this formula could not be applied this way directly as it considers only one expression value per tissue. On the contrary, the dataset contained several samples per tissue and significant differences were present between the number of samples available for each tissue. Therefore, the formula was applied for every lncRNA but considering N as the total number of samples (161). The expression values of every lncRNA were scaled and centred prior to applying the formula. Finally, lncRNAs with *tau* values above 0.7 were considered to be tissue-specific.

A Spearman correlation analysis was performed for every lncRNA versus the expression of all the protein-coding genes. A protein-coding gene was considered significantly correlated if a correlation value over 0.8 was obtained. GOSeq R package was used to perform the functional enrichment for each lncRNA using a built-in matrix based on correlated and non-correlated protein-coding genes. P-values were adjusted using the Benjamini & Hochberg method and only p-values under 0.05 were considered significant. Blast2GO [64] was used to create some combined graphs to highlight the functions most widely shared across the lncRNAs. The described approach was followed for both tissue-specific and non-tissue-specific lncRNAs.

5.3.2 Results

Bias detection and count normalisation

Different density plots were made to measure the expression ranges of both protein-coding genes and long non-coding RNAs. As previously reported, both transcript types have very different expression ranges. A scatter plot (Figure 5.1) was created to explore the differences between two random protein-coding and two long non-coding RNA genes. Expression values of protein-coding genes are almost two orders of magnitude higher than long non-coding RNAs.

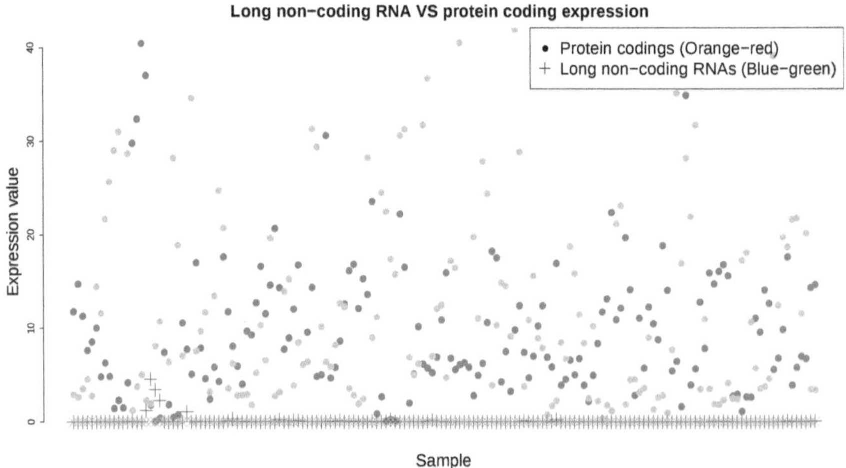

Figure 5.1: Expression values of two random protein-coding and two long non-coding RNA genes to show that, in general, the expression values of protein-coding genes are almost two orders of magnitude higher than long non-coding RNAs.

Principal Component Analysis (PCA) was performed for the protein-coding genes and long non-coding genes using the log10 of the counts from the previous step to measure any possible bias (Figure 5.2).

As a strong laboratory bias was detected in the data that required correction, we used ASCA-genes to correct and normalise the data. Moreover, due to the need for comparing the expression of genes regardless of the sequencing depths, the count matrix was further normalised using the quantile normalisation method (Figure 5.3).

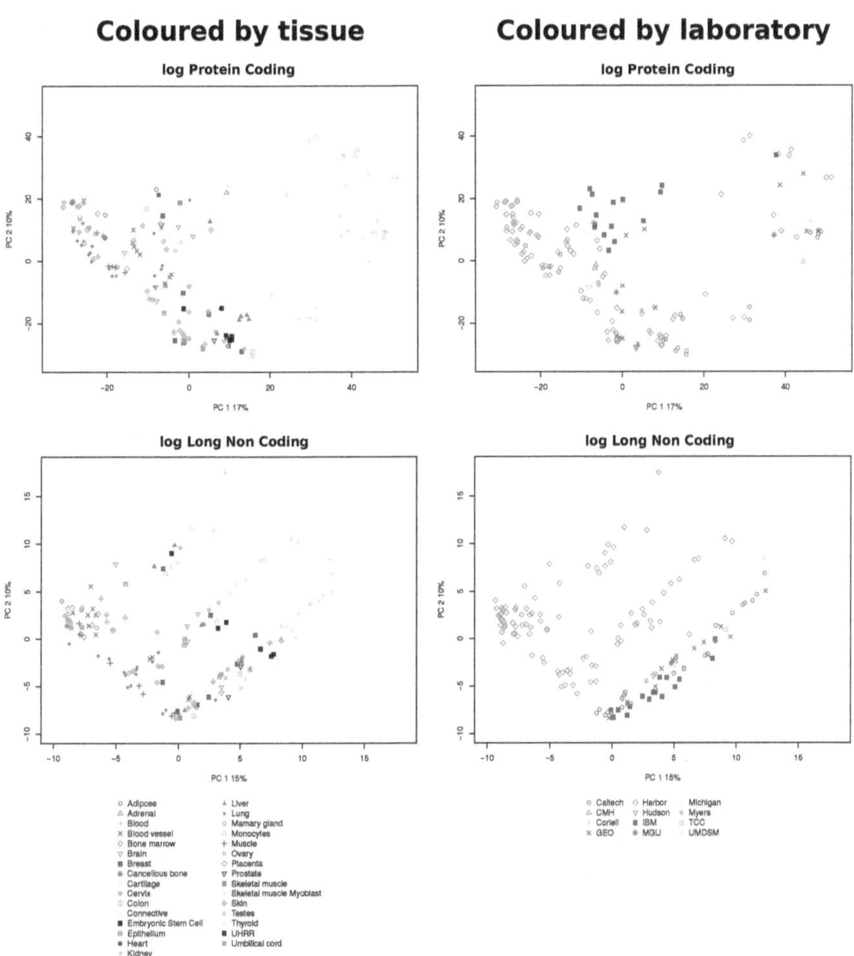

Figure 5.2: PCA of coding and long-non coding RNAs across a wide range of tissues. Counts were corrected by sequencing depth.

Functional annotation

As seen in Figure 5.1, the expression of lncRNAs is in general low, being some orders of magnitude lower than protein-coding genes. This is one of the ncRNA features that makes this kind of transcripts especially difficult to characterise.

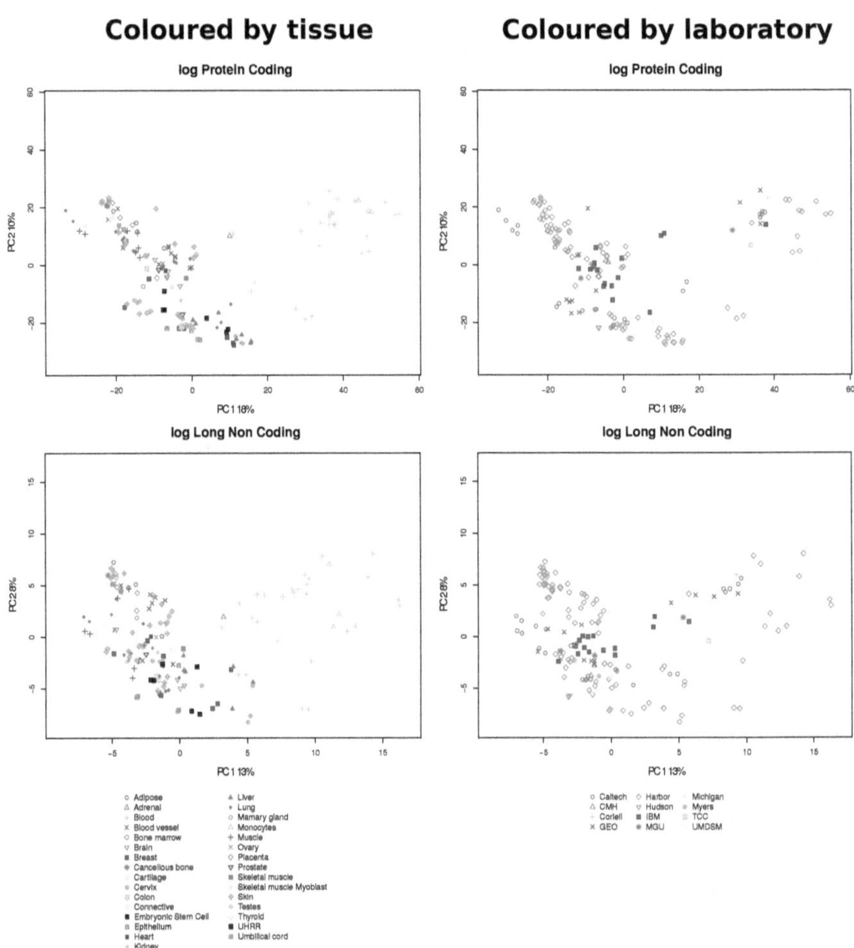

Figure 5.3: PCA of coding and long-non coding RNAs across a wide range of tissues. Data were batch-corrected and normalised using the quantile normalisation approach.

A guilty-by-association approach was followed to perform the functional annotation of lncRNAs. Following this approach, a lncRNA will be annotated with the Gene Ontology (GO) terms the correlated protein-coding genes are enriched with. Although the guilty-by-association approach has often been used to characterise novel genes, in this case, we face a data analysis challenge due to the different order of magnitude in the expression of coding and non-coding genes, and also the fact that most lncRNAs are expressed only in a few tissues, while coding genes are more prevalent across tissues. This fact required specific correlation strategies.

First, different density plots were made for both lncRNAs and protein-coding gene expression values to define a point at which they could be considered expressed (Figure 5.4). The threshold value used was 1, so all protein-coding genes and lncRNAs with a lower expression across all the samples were filtered out. This first filter was passed by 4552 out of the 13047 lncRNAs and 17907 out of the 20203 protein-coding genes.

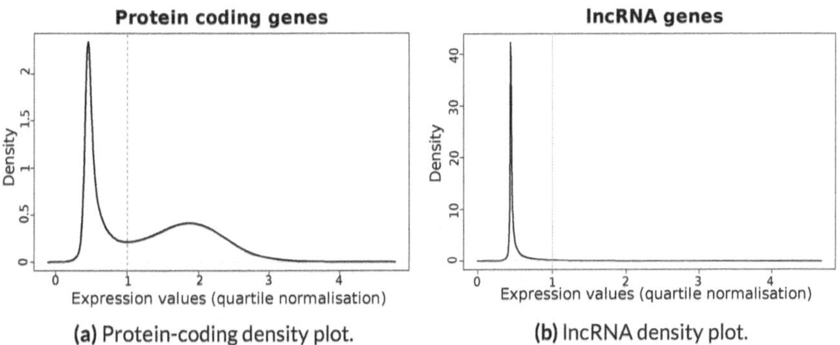

(a) Protein-coding density plot. (b) lncRNA density plot.

Figure 5.4: Density plots applied over the expression values using quantile normalisation. Red line indicates the minimum threshold used for both biotypes to consider them as expressed.

Correlation calculations are usually a good approach when working with many data with values over 0. However, lncRNA expression tend to be really low due to being expressed only in some specific tissues, so using a correlation approach was not the best decision in this case. To address this issue, we used the *tau* formula [5.1][63] to create two different groups of lncRNAs, that is, tissue-specific and non-tissue-specific lncRNAs.

After applying the formula, lncRNAs with *tau* values above 0.7 were considered to be tissue-specific (3542 out of 4552).

Just as important as knowing whether they are tissue-specific or not is knowing the tissues in which they are overexpressed. For this reason, those tissues with an expression 3 times above the interquartile range were considered for all the tissue-specific genes. For the cases in which replicates were available, only the tissues in which at least 75% of the replicates fulfilled the previous threshold were considered. However, there were a few lncRNAs that, using these criteria, were not associated to any overexpressed tissue despite having a *tau* over the 0.7 threshold. These lncRNAs were finally considered as non-specific. Figure 5.5 shows the number of tissues in which the tissue-specific lncRNAs were specific after applying the latest constraint. 15% of the lncRNAs (pale blue) considered tissue-specific in the first instance were discarded because it was not possible to find a single tissue in which they could be considered overexpressed. However, the vast majority of the tissue-specific lncRNAs were considered specific in more than 1 tissue. A ranking containing the most over-expressed tissues within the tissue-specific lncRNAs was also performed, showing Hmncpb, Lymphoma, White blood cells, Skeletal muscle and Lymphoblastoid - 79 year in the top 5. LncRNAs were found specific in 95 out of the 162 different samples as shown in Figure 5.6.

A Spearman correlation analysis was performed for every lncRNAs versus the expression of all the protein-coding genes. Functional enrichment was performed using GOSeq R package and their p-values were adjusted using the Benjamini & Hochberg method. Only 374 GO terms in total were obtained for the non-tissue-specific lncRNAs whereas a total of 202818 were obtained for the tissue-specific lncRNAs.

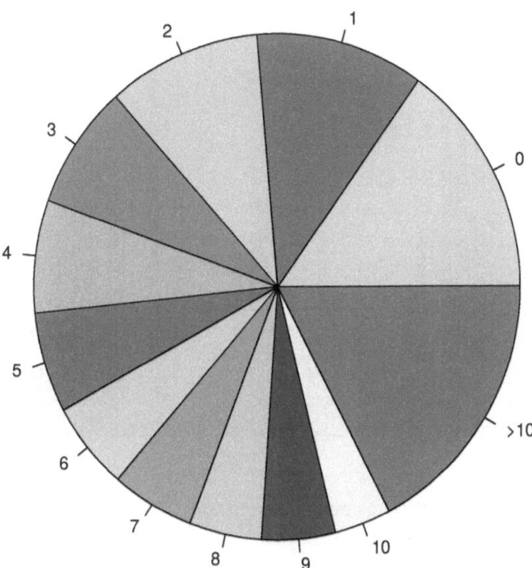

Figure 5.5: Number of tissues the lncRNAs are specific in.

Blast2GO [64] was used to create some combined graphs highlighting the most widely functions shared across the lncRNAs. Figures 5.7 and 5.8 show the biological processes and molecular functions of the tissue-specific lncRNAs and figure 5.9 shows the biological process from the extracted GO terms of the non-tissue-specific lncRNAs. The darker the colour the more significant the functions are.

Tissue-specific lncRNAs seem to be related with RNA and DNA binding processes, signalling, immune system response and basic cellular processes among others. Non-tissue-specific lncRNAs seem to have less generic functions, mainly focusing on cellular processes such as G-protein coupled receptor signalling pathway and the detection of chemical stimulus involved in sensory perception of bitter

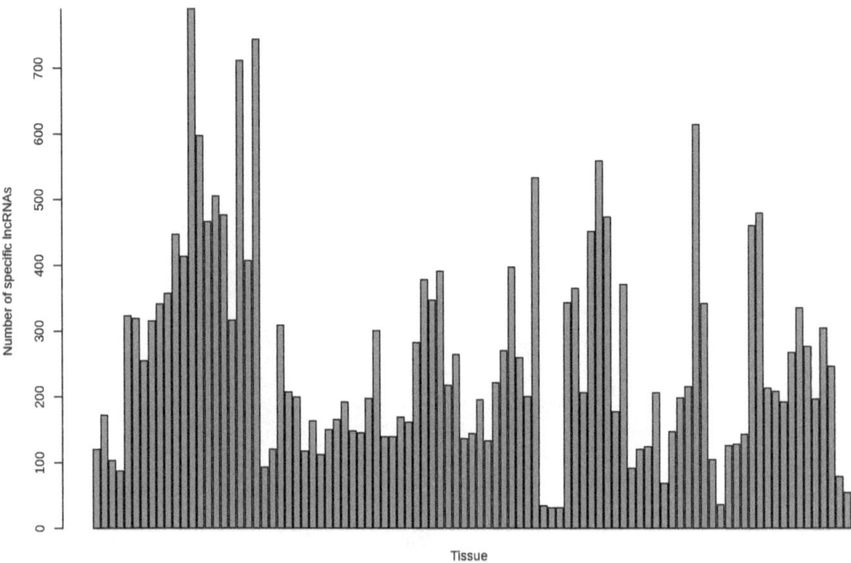

Figure 5.6: The number of lncRNAs specific per tissue. Tissues that were not specific of any lncRNAs were discarded from the representation.

taste. However, differences in how specific the functions between tissue-specific and non-tissue-specific lncRNAs are mainly due to the important difference in the number of GO terms obtained for each, so the functions of non-tissue-specific lncRNAs should be taken with caution.

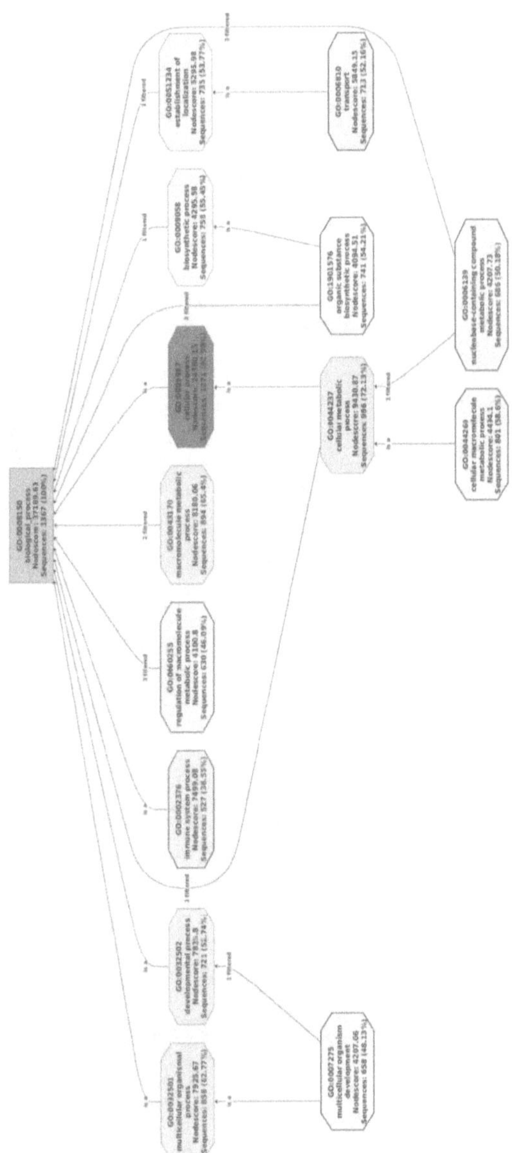

Figure 5.7: Biological processes of tissue-specific lncRNAs.

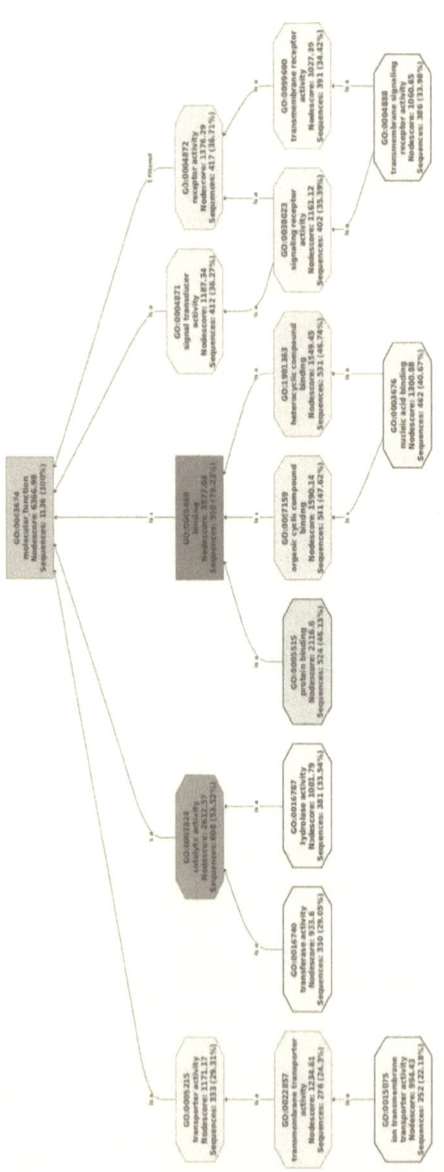

Figure 5.8: Molecular functions of tissue-specific lncRNAs.

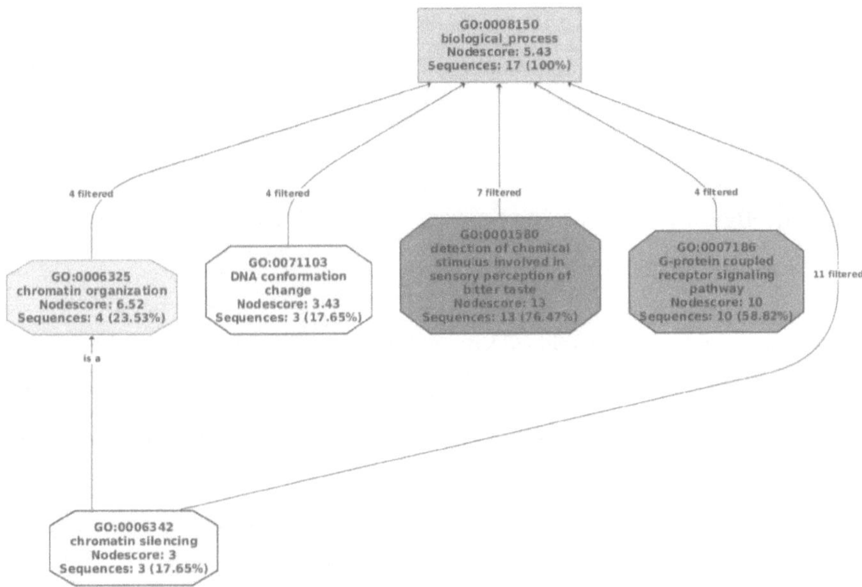

Figure 5.9: Biological processes of non-tissue-specific lncRNAs.

5.3.3 Conclusion

LncRNAs are known to act as important regulators. However, little is still known regarding their functions. Here we present a new approach for the functional characterisation of lncRNAs where we analysed RNA-Seq data extracted from public repositories gathering samples from very different tissues. A guilty-by-association approach was used to obtain a final list of GO terms for each possible lncRNA. Finally, tissue-specific and non-tissue-specific lncRNAs generic functions were extracted.

Though data was cleaned and normalised as much as possible, final data was still far from perfect. Besides, most of the known statistical approaches do not behave well when little or no expression is found in genes, a common condition of lncRNAs. Given those facts and despite trying other statistical methods before the one finally exposed, we can conclude the results obtained through the analysis were not completely satisfactory.

5.4 spongeScan: A web for detecting microRNA binding elements in lncRNA sequences

Non-coding RNAs such as microRNAs (miRNAs) are now well established as important biological regulators. In particular, miRNAs act both to destabilise the transcripts they bind to or to inhibit their translation. Under certain conditions, miRNAs can also activate translation or regulate the transcription. The interaction with their target genes depends on many factors such as the abundance of both miRNAs and target mRNAs, the affinity of the interactions, etc. This binding event is mediated by a protein complex that recruits the mature miRNA to its target transcript and guide its binding through base-pair complementarity, between the miRNA "seed sequence" (6-8 nucleotides long) in its 5'-end and its target site in the 3'UTR of the transcript sequence. While many features have been associated with active miRNA binding sites, it is clear that complementarity is most important at the 'seed' region of the miRNA, i.e. nucleotides 2–8 of the mature miRNA [65]. Complementarity between the rest of the miRNA and the target sequence is usually high. Once bound, miRNAs can negatively influence their translation or stimulate the active deadenylation and decapping of the target transcript with other factors, causing the degradation of the mRNA. Many methods have been published to detect possible miRNA target sites (e.g. TargetScan, miRanda and PicTar [66, 67, 68]), usually searching for high-complementarity, seed complementarity, conservation and other features in the 3'UTRs of mRNA sequences. More recently, it has been demonstrated that the activity of some miRNAs may be regulated through so-called competitive endogenous RNAs (ceRNAs) [27]. These are non-coding transcripts that harbour miRNA response elements (MREs) where miRNAs bind. If these ceRNAs possess many MREs and are expressed at high enough levels they can sequester circulating miRNAs, thus reducing their number and activity on target mRNAs.

Identification of ceRNAs and their target miRNAs is a challenge. Given that ceRNAs are usually ncRNAs and that they are likely to possess an abundance of putative binding sites for miRNAs, regular prediction tools that seek for single miRNA binding site are not optimised to detect ceRNAs candidates. AGO CLIP-seq, as well as RNA-Seq, has been used to propose thousands of lncRNA–miRNA interactions [69, 70] but these methods are restricted by the availability of such data for specific organisms and cell types. We sought to address these limitations by developing a novel, sequence-based, algorithm designed for the detection of MREs in non-coding transcripts that would be potentially applicable to any organism where sequence data exist.

5.4.1 Architecture

spongeScan has been designed using a client-server architecture and can be divided into three different modules: 1) the prediction algorithm, written in C++; 2) the client, a web application interface built using the Sencha framework and developed to launch new predictions and to allow the dynamic visualisation of the results; and 3) the server side, containing a full set of web services to allow all possible interactions with the client part built using the Flask library from Python, as well as a NoSQL database to store and query the prediction results using MongoDB.

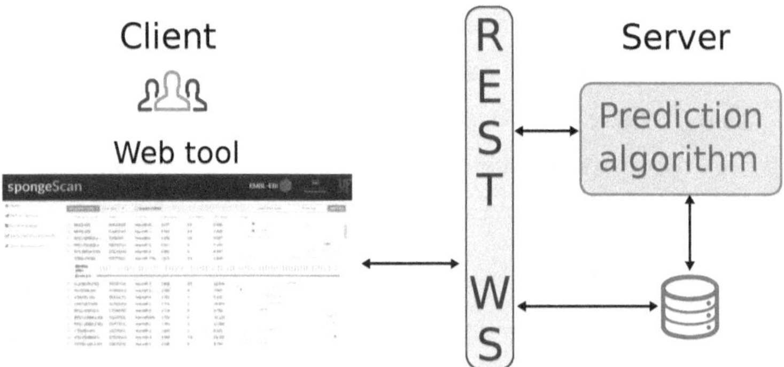

Figure 5.10: spongeScan architecture.

5.4.2   The algorithm

spongeScan is a web resource to find highly enriched MRE binding sites in lncRNAs. Users must provide the lncRNA transcript sequences in a FASTA file. These sequences can be automatically retrieved by spongeScan from any release and species available at Ensembl [71] or be directly uploaded by the user. Additionally, an annotation GTF file is necessary. This file is used to obtain the biotype of the transcripts to filter out those that are not lncRNAs, if any.

spongeScan looks for sequence complementarity between any possible k-mer of 6, 7 or 8 nucleotides in each lncRNA and identifies if any of these enriched k-mers corresponds to a known miRNAs seed sequence. To do this, the user has to indicate the species being analysed and spongeScan will look for the corresponding miRNAs in the miRBase database [72] automatically at runtime. Retrieved miRNAs are then filtered to keep the canonical seeds of 6, 7 and 8 nucleotides of only experimentally validated miRNAs (Figure 5.11).

For each possible k-mer, spongeScan scans for matches using sliding windows of varying sizes ranging from 50 bps to 1 kb in steps of 50 bps allowing up to one G:U

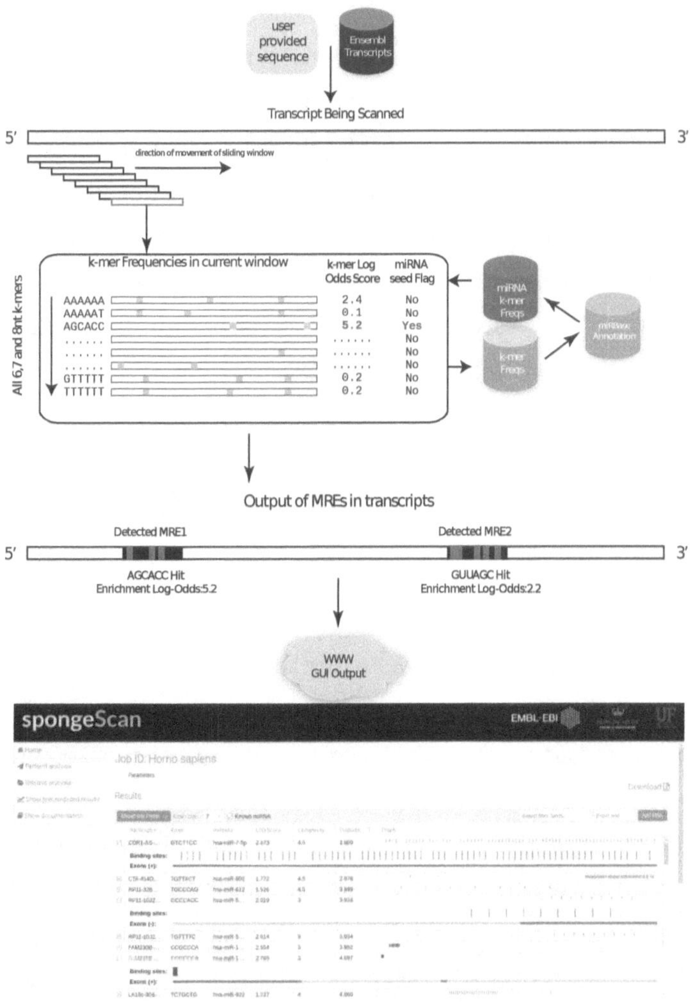

Figure 5.11: Flowchart showing the main strategy behind the spongeScan application. K-mers of 6, 7 and 8 nucleotides are searched for by using sliding windows of different sizes. Different k-mer frequencies are obtained for each pair k-mer – lncRNA. Highly enriched k-mers are reported and checked for correspondence with a miRNA canonical seed. Pairwise predictions are then represented in spongeScan.

wobble (Figure 5.11). This varying sliding window approach allows selecting the window size that returns the highest number of matches, thereby allowing for flexibility in the k-mer distribution. From k-mer frequencies, we compute a Log-Odds score (LOD, 5.2) to identify and report highly enriched k-mers for each lncRNA. The formula below is used to obtain the maximum number of matches for which significant pairing between a k-mer and lncRNA are found across all the sliding windows. This is compared to the maximum number of occurrences of that same k-mer in all other lncRNA sequences. This is calculated for all the possible window sizes and reports the one with the highest LOD.

$$LOD_{kmer,transcript} = log\left(\frac{max(occur_{kmer,transcript})}{\sum_{i=0}^{N}max(occur_{kmer,i})} \times N\right) \qquad (5.2)$$

A dispersion score 5.3 is also calculated for every pair to evaluate the clustering of binding sites. As we are trying different window sizes, the maximum number of matches should change accordingly. For instance, if two matches of a k-mer in a window size of 50 are detected and these are approximately equally distributed, we should expect four matches to be found using a window size of 100, etc. For this reason, we build a vector containing the maximum number of occurrences normalised by the window size used and calculate the standard deviation. This value is what we called dispersion score. The lower this value is, the most equally distributed the miRNA seed matches are. This parameter allows to make hypothesis on the distribution pattern on MREs along the ceRNAs. Known ceRNAs tend to have equally spaced MREs that would facilitate multiple miRNA binding [27], which implies a low dispersion score.

$$x_i = \forall_{50:50}^{1000} \frac{w\_size}{max_{occur}}$$

$$DS_{kmer,transcript} = \sqrt{\frac{\sum(x_i - \bar{x})}{N - 1}} \tag{5.3}$$

Finally, a complexity score 5.4 is calculated for all the k-mers not matching with any known miRNA canonical seed, and k-mers with low complexity scores are filtered out. The formula measures the number of single nucleotides and di-nucleotides, i.e. a k-mer containing AAAAAA would be $(6 - 6) \times 0.5 + 1 \times 0.5 = 0.5$, whereas ATGCTA would be $(6 - 2) \times 0.5 + 5 \times 0.5 = 4.5$. This score is used to filter out low complexity k-mers that may return unspecific binding.

$$CS_{kmer} = (kmer\_length - max(A|C|T|G)) \times 0.5 + different\_dinucleotides \times 0.5 \tag{5.4}$$

The default thresholds for the Log-Odd score, dispersion and complexity scores are 1, 10 and 4, respectively. However, these values can be modified in the web application. For example, a higher LOD score and lower dispersion score would select lncRNAs with a higher number of MREs and more evenly distributed sites. Other additional and adjustable arguments are the total number of binding sites detected for a pair lncRNA:k-mer. By default, the application will only report pairs where more than 20 putative binding sites have been found for a k-mer in a lncRNA sequence. In contrast to other algorithms such as DIANA-microT [69], that use PAR-CLIP[2] data to identify putative MREs, spongeScan exclusively relies on sequence data and bases its scoring system in the number of matched sites and their distribution along the lncRNA sequence. This favours, on one hand, the de-

---

[2]Photoactivatable ribonucleoside-enhanced crosslinking and immunoprecipitation (PAR-CLIP) is a biochemical method for identifying the binding sites of cellular RNA-binding proteins (RBPs) and microRNA-containing ribonucleoprotein complexes (miRNPs).

tection of ceRNAs where miRNA sequestration can occur at multiple sites, and on the other hand, allows application of the algorithm to any organism.

Once computations are completed, spongeScan displays identified lncRNA:k-mer pairs in a tabular format, where each row represents a different match. Results for k-mers of 6, 7 or 8 nucleotides are kept separately and the user can switch between them. Additionally, the results distinguish between k-mers matching known miRNAs or unknown k-mers. The results table has up to 22 different columns containing different information or statistics regarding the pairing. This table can be sorted and filtered by any of the available fields. A graphical representation of the lncRNA sequence showing the positions where the k-mer is found is also included. Matched locations can be clicked to open an integrated genome viewer [73] for closer examination of the binding sites. Additionally, if expression data have been provided, a bar plot showing the expression of the selected lncRNA and miRNA(s) will be displayed. The complete manual of the web application can be found online:

5.4.3   Web services

The core of the application is on the server side. The communication between the client side (web application) and the server is made via RESTful web services [3]. For this purpose, nine different web services have been implemented. These web services could be divided as follows:

Job submission

---

[3]Representational State Transfer (REST) is a software architectural style that defines a set of constraints to be used for creating Web services. Web services that conform to the REST architectural style (RESTful Web services) provide interoperability between computer systems on the Internet using Uniform Resource Identifiers (URIs), typically links on the Web.

/submit(POST)

This is the web service used to perform new predictions. The different arguments, as well as the fasta, GTF and expression files are sent using the POST HTTP method.

Job information retrieval

/getArguments/<job_id>(GET)

This web service is used to retrieve the different arguments that were used to perform the prediction of the job id *job_id*.

/getJob/<job_id>/<kmer_size>/<known> (GET)

This web service is called to obtain the prediction results and to be able to load the grid table form the web application. Basically, it will need to get the job id, the size of the kmers (*kmer_size*) and whether the results must be from kmers with miRNA canonical seed matches or not (*known*). Besides, additional arguments are given for table navigation purposes.

/jobStatus/<job_id> (GET)

This web service is called every time a user asks for the retrieval of a job. Basically, this will inform the web application whether the job with the given job id has been finished and the results can be checked or not.

/getKmers/<job_id>/<positions>/<kmer_size> (GET)

Called to obtain the different k-mers of a concrete kmer size within the given genomic positions. These positions are given in positions with the following format: chr1:1-100,chr1:101-200 for example. This is used to represent these k-mers in the genomic viewer.

/getExpression/<job_id>/<gene_ids> (GET)

The web service is used to obtain the expression values of the genes given in *gene_ids* of a concrete job. This will be used to represent those expression values using bar plots.

/download/<job_id>/<kmer_size>/<known> (GET)

This web service is called to obtain a CSV file containing all the predictions of a given job, with the k-mers of 6, 7 or 8 nucleotides and with miRNA seed matches or not.

Auxiliar web services

/getEnsemblCDNAs (GET)

This web service is used to load the ncRNA fasta files available from Ensembl. The release and species can be supplied to obtain the final results using the GET HTTP method.

/getEnsemblGTFs (GET)

The same way as the previous web service, this one will be checking for the possible GTF files available in Ensembl for a given species and release.

All the web services, except the one that returns the CSV file with the results, return a JSON file format that will be parsed and interpreted properly by the web application.

5.4.4 *Web application*

The web application has been developed using the version 5.1.1 of the Sencha Ext JS framework. The look of the web application is shown in Figure 5.12. The menu is located on the left side of the application.

spongeScan could be divided into two different sections: 1) new job submission section where the researchers will upload or select the species they would like to

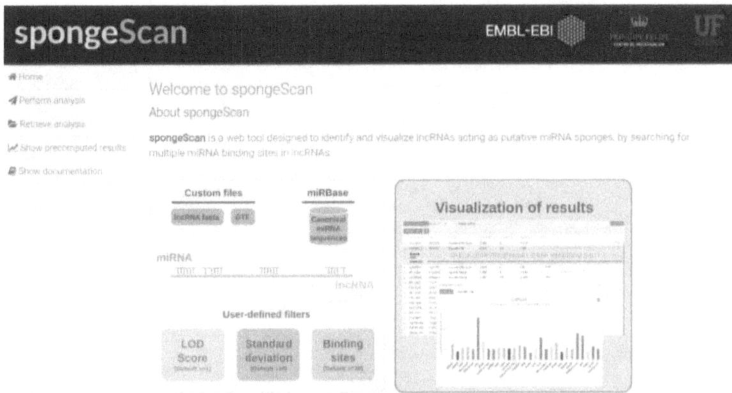

Figure 5.12: Main view of the spongeScan web application.

explore; and 2) the representation of the results obtained after running the prediction algorithm under the user requirements.

5.4.4.1 New analysis

Performing new predictions are really straightforward using spongeScan. To do so, the user will have to click the *Perform analysis* link from the left bar of the menu and the form from Figure 5.13 will be displayed.

The user will have to choose the GTF annotation file as well as the corresponding lncRNA transcript fasta file to run the computations. To do so, spongeScan shows all the available GTF and transcript files for any species available in Ensembl since release 50. Moreover, as the user might also be interested in using their own custom annotation and transcript files, an option to upload their own custom files have been added. This is done in points 1 and 2 of Figure 5.13.

spongeScan will look for putative miRNA binding sites across the lncRNA sequences. Therefore, miRNA sequences must also be obtained for computational

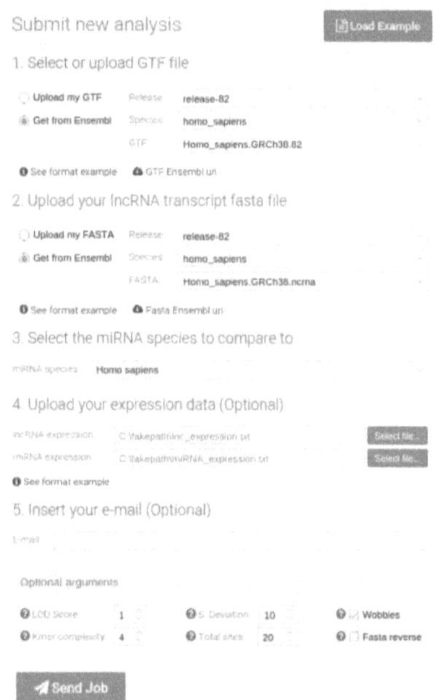

Figure 5.13: Form to perform a new prediction analysis with the default example options loaded.

purposes. In point 3, all available species with miRNA information in miRBase database are loaded. The user will have to select the species where the canonical seed sequences will be obtained from.

The user might also have expression data that would like to upload in the application (point 4). This expression data has to be uploaded using a predefined format as it will be represented using two different levels, per tissue and per replicate. The first three lines of the file must contain the tags *Description*, *Tissue* and *Sample* followed by the format of the expression values, the tissues and the samples or replicates used respectively. The following lines will contain the expression value in a tabular mode, one per gene. A basic representation of the format is shown below:

```
#Description FPKM values
#Tissue Epithelium Epithelium Adipose Adrenal
#Sample A549_Rp1-2 A549_Rp3 Adipose Ag04450
ENSG00000242268 0.39 0.41 0.41 0.43
ENSG00000249023 0.43 0.43 0.44 0.46

...
```

Once a new prediction has been run by the user using the send job button, a random and unique job id will be associated. This job id will be shown automatically to the user once the job has been requested and will be necessary to recover and check the results of the prediction. Additionally, the user might want to insert its e-mail address. This way, an e-mail will be sent at the beginning of the job with the job information, at the end of the job notifying the user the possibility of checking the results and another one in case of failure at any point of the prediction.

Finally, the parameters that will be used when performing the predictions can be also modified by the user. This allows more flexibility to change the prediction criteria.

5.4.4.2   Results visualisation

To recover the results of any prediction, the user will have to click the *Retrieve analysis* link at the left bar of the application and input the corresponding job id.

5.4.5   Example data set

spongeScan contains an example data set consisting of precomputed results for the MRE search algorithm in human lncRNAs together with gene expression information for these and miRNAs across several tissues obtained by metanalysis of publicly available RNA-Seq data. The human MRE search was done using the *Homo sapiens* ncRNA fasta file from Ensembl release 82 and the corresponding GTF annotation file. Algorithm parameters were set to k-mer complexity scores > 4, LOD > 1, standard deviation < 30, minimum number of predicted = 2 and allowing for one G:U wobble.

To obtain gene expression values for ncRNAs and miRNAs, 206 human RNA-Seq data sets were downloaded from SRA and ENCODE [13] corresponding to several healthy tissues and cell lines, while 12 miRNA-Seq data sets were found for the same tissues. RNA-Seq data were analyzed with standard procedures [74], using Tophat [75] as mapper and htseq-count [76] as quantification tool. Quantification was obtained for a total of 13,047 lncRNAs and 1,548 microRNAs, and values were uploaded into spongeScan.

When ranking results by LOD the known sponge CDR1-AS acting on mir-7 was one of the top 50 hits and the absolute top hit when ranked by dispersion score (Figure 5.14A). Visualisation of gene expression data reveals that CDR1-AS is preferentially expressed in brain tissue (Figure 5.14B), as previously described [27]. To further evaluate whether a sequestration effect was happening, we analysed the potential effect of predicted lncRNAs with multiple MREs in sequestering to explain the down-regulatory effect of bound miRNAs over their target genes, as previously described [27]. We obtained target genes for miRNAs in predicted pairs from TargetScan and compared their expression levels in tissues with or without the expression of the putative sponge, using a paired t-test. Once more, this analysis indicated that in all tissue comparisons (100%) expression of mir-7 targets was upregulated when CDR1-AS was expressed (Figure 5.14C). Unfortunately, not enough matching tissue data were available for similar analyses in other putative sponges.

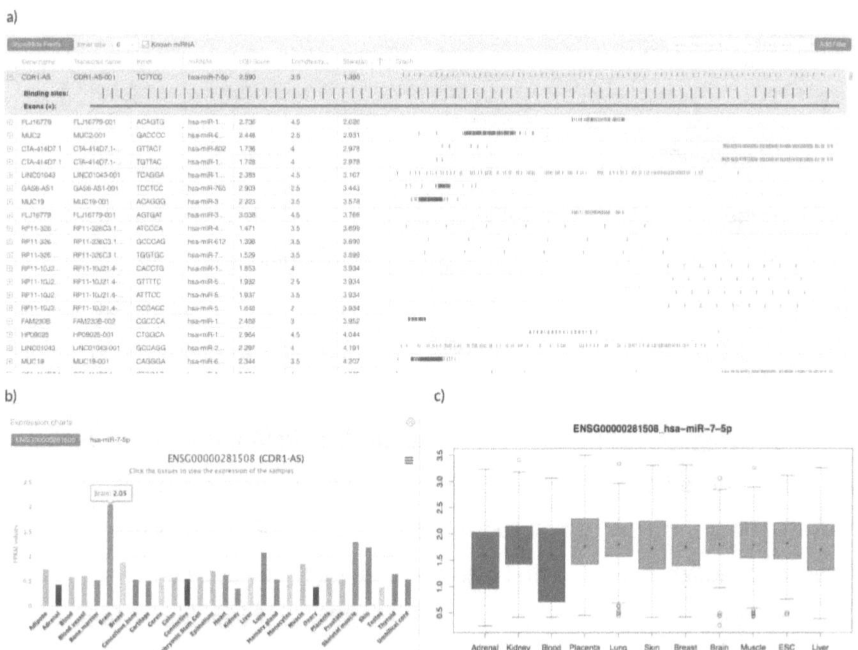

Figure 5.14: spongeScan output generated for the example data set. (A) Table showing pairwise enrichments of miRNA canonical seeds in lncRNA sequences. This view only shows a few of the total possible columns containing data and scores. (B) Expression data representation for the first pair CDR1-AS and miR-7-5p. The expression data are grouped by tissue and, when clicked, it will show the expression of all the samples in the tissue. (C) Expression levels of mRNA targets of miR-7 for different tissues as a function of the CDR1-AS expression. Red box-plots correspond to tissues where the lncRNA is not significantly expressed, whereas the green colour indicates expression of the lncRNA in the tissue.

Finally, we compared our results with the list of lncRNA–miRNA interactions available at lncBase [69]. lncBase provides a prediction score for human lncRNA–miRNA interactions based on different evidence sources. We have observed that validated lncRNA–microRNA pairs in this database usually have scores from 0.4 to 1.0. We searched the top 100 results on our human example data and found that most (81%) of our predictions were in the lncBase, having an average score of 0.84 in this database [77], what supports our prediction results with an independent resource.

5.4.6   Conclusions

We describe spongeScan, a novel web application and algorithm able to identify putative miRNA binding patterns across lncRNA sequences. The algorithm is based on sequence complementarity and allows flexibility for the user to customise the choice of parameters. The possibility of adding expression data to the prediction representation in the web tool greatly facilitates downstream functional analysis. spongeScan differs from other lncRNA–miRNA interactions prediction sites that utilize CLIP-seq data [69, 70] in allowing massive searches on user-provided data and in being available for any organism with sequence information. To our knowledge, this is the first web resource that provides a universal searchable engine for the identification of putative lncRNAs with multiple MREs. Overall, we believe spongeScan will be extremely useful for the discovery of crosstalk between lncRNAs and miRNAs.

## Chapter 6

General discussion and conclusions

6.1 Overview

This book focuses on the analysis of gene expression data provided by current high throughput sequencing approaches. Specifically, the aim was to develop new bioinformatic tools that would cover existing gaps acknowledged by the scientific community regarding data analysis and integration of omics data, specifically in the area of transcriptomics. In particular, I have studied the role of good quality controls on the analysis of RNA-seq count data and collaborated in the implementation of an R package called NOISeq that contains a full suite of diagnostic plots and a broad range of different functions to assess quality and normalise data. I have also contributed to the SEQC project through the study of the reproducibility of RNA-Seq technology under different conditions. Motivated by the need to perform integrative analysis in multiomics projects, I implemented a Python script named RGmatch for matching genomic regions to the nearest exons, transcripts and/or genes that can be highly customised to meet user needs. Finally, I studied the importance of lncRNAs and created an algorithm to functionally characterise them on a global scale. Within this area, we created a new web tool called spongeScan to specifically detect lncRNAs that could be acting as miRNA sponges, therefore inhibiting their functions.

6.2 Discussion and conclusions

In chapter 3, I contributed to the quality control of RNA-seq count data by collaborating in the implementation of an R package called NOISeq, designed for the exploratory analysis and differential expression of genes for RNA-Seq, which was later published in Bioconductor. The tool supports up to six different exploratory plots to analyse different aspects of the quality of the data and implements a nonparametric approach for the differential expression analysis. The development of the R package was guided by two different principles:

- reusability: NOISeq uses the *ExpressionSet* S4 class to store all the relevant information to be used by the different metric tools and implements new S4 classes where specific needs not covered by other available classes are required;

- modularity: NOISeq code is decomposed into different separated pieces that could perform different analysis while reusing the same main input object.

Reproducibility of RNA-Seq technology was also assessed in collaboration with the SEQC study. Bias effects were detected when comparing results of the analysis across different laboratories. In this case, we demonstrated that a major factor responsible for these biases is sequencing depth. Indeed, we clearly showed that the higher the sequencing depth the highest the number of detected differentially expressed genes without a clear trend towards a saturation point. Despite normalisation by sequencing depth is strongly necessary, this correction did not still completely mitigate the biases introduced by the fact of having samples with large sequencing depth differences. These observations have two practical implications: firstly, in terms of experimental design, all samples included in a comparison should be sequenced at the same depth to avoid confounding experimental factors. Secondly, reporting of DE analysis findings should always indicate the level of sequencing at which they were found, as differential expression calls are not absolute but dependent on sequencing depth.

Another aspect studied was the usage of replicates in an RNA-Seq analysis. Replica sets are strongly recommended for new transcript detection, especially for the detection of transcripts with a low expression level. Approaches that filter out these transcripts are also recommended as they reduce the noise and spare statistical power. Highly-expressed transcripts, on the contrary, seemed to be fairly consistent across replicates. Replicates can also be beneficial for junction detection analysis. Given our results, we strongly support that a minimum of 2-3 replicates should be enough for the detection of highly expressed genes. However, we would suggest using at least 5 replicates for the detection of genes with low expression.

In chapter 4, a new tool for matching genomic regions and genes is presented, RGmatch. Despite the tool covering only a small part of the integration process pipeline, this step is essential to assist the integrative analysis of multiomics data as genome localisation data needs to be linked to expressed genes. Therefore, RGmatch can be used to integrate very different assays, such as ChIP-seq, DNase-seq, ATAC-seq, all different types of DNA methylation studies, and even Hi-C data, with each other and also with gene expression. The main benefits of the tool developed in comparison to others available are:

- user-friendly command-line tool;

- easy integration into any analysis pipeline;

- the user chooses the association resolution level (gene, transcript or exon);

- fully customisable tool in which the user can define the conflict resolution rules as well as custom lengths for TSS, TTS and PROMOTER regions;

- no species limitation. The tool can be run over any species as long as an annotation GTF is present;

- the script has an insignificant memory and time execution footprint.

These benefits have already been exploited. We easily integrated RGmatch into the PaintOmics 3 tool to allow mapping of chromatin data into KEGG pathways defined by their participating genes [78]. Specifically, RGmatch is used to link any type of BED data to genes and subsequently to the pathways they are involved in.

Finally, in chapter 5 we focused on the functional characterisation of lncRNAs. To do so, RNA-Seq data from public repositories was downloaded and analysed. As described previously in many publications, we observed that lncRNAs are extremely tissue-specific. Our analyses re-confirmed that the expression of lncRNAs is several orders of magnitude lower than protein-coding genes. These two facts make the functional characterisation of lncRNAs a difficult task because they don't fulfil the basic criteria needed to use many known statistical methods. During this analysis we evidenced the huge challenge in the harmonisation of public heterogeneous data, mainly because of the data quality, laboratory batch effects and sequencing depth differences. Given the large heterogeneous dataset, we opted for performing a guilty-by-association study in which we searched for protein-coding genes co-expressed with lncRNA genes, and assumed the lncRNAs are implicated in the regulation of the related protein-coding gene functions. We made a distinction between tissue and non-tissue-specific lncRNAs although not many GO terms could be extracted for the latter, possibly due to the difficulty in establishing meaningful correlations with only a few tissues. The results showed that most of the tissue-specific lncRNAs were related to RNA and DNA binding processes, signalling, immune system response and basic cellular processes among others, whereas non-tissue-specific lncRNAs were related to less generic functions, such as chromatin organisation or DNA conformation change. We acknowledge that these results should be taken cautiously. After completion of this work other studies have attempted a similar approach using thousands of samples and created a database containing all this information. However, given the complexity of the problem, their goal is to store the results of many of these analyses performed over different RNA-Seq datasets to make a proper validation.

In the last part of the chapter, we also show the development of a new web application and algorithm for the identification of lncRNAs acting as miRNA sponges. Many publications have shown the significance of the detection of these lncRNAs as they play an important role in different forms of cancer. Given the relevance, we implemented a user-friendly web application to help identify putative miRNA binding elements in lncRNA sequences. A sequence complementarity algorithm is run and several scores are calculated (LOD score, complexity score and dispersity score) for every possible miRNA - lncRNA pair. The higher the LOD score the more likely the miRNA can be exclusively sequestered by that lncRNA. The higher the complexity score the more complex the miRNA sequence is (less repetitive nucleotides) and the lower the dispersity score, the more homogeneously distributed the binding locations are. User-defined thresholds for the three scores are used to create the final report of putative miRNA sponges. Additionally, expression data can be also inputted and automatically plotted for each reported pair to help researchers decide which of them can be trusted candidates. The benefits of the tool in comparison to others available are:

- inclusion of expression data to better identify candidates;

- massive searches on user-provided data;

- availability of the tool for any annotated organism.

6.3   Reach and relevance

The relevance of this book is justified in the following points:

- The tools and methods presented in this book were developed under the framework of four international research projects: TRANSPAT (Development of transcriptional networks regulating virulence in filamentous fungi from RNA-seq data), PIB2010AR (Genomics and transcriptomics of dexotification pathways in Drosophila and Development of Computational Approaches for the characterization), STATegra (User-driven development of statistical methods for experimental planning, data gathering, and integrative analysis of Next Generation Sequencing, proteomics and metabolomics data) and Annot-lincRNA (functional annotation of long-non-coding RNAs).

- The tools developed, NOISeq Bioconductor R package, RGmatch and spongeScan, are all freely available to the scientific community. Furthermore, RGmatch has been integrated as the main "region to gene matcher" in the PaintOmics 3 [78] web tool.

- This work was developed with the main goal of having an impact and being useful for the scientific community. This fact is reflected by the publications of most of these results in highly impact and relevant to the field journals.